My frame was not hidden from You when I was being made in secret, intricately woven in the depths of the earth. Your eyes beheld my unformed substance.
Psalms 139: 15–16, New Revised Standard Version, Harper Collins

To my parents, Modupe and Olatunji, and Madam Sarah Ogbede with thanks

For Elsevier

Senior Commissioning Editor: Sarena Wolfaard
Project Development Manager: Dinah Thom
Project Manager: Joannah Duncan
Design Direction: Judith Wright

Obstetrics and Gynaecology Ultrasound

A self-assessment guide

Oluwakemi O. Ola-Ojo MSc GDU BSc DCR

Senior 1 Radiographer/Ultrasonographer, London, UK

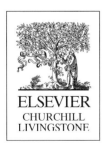

ELSEVIER
CHURCHILL
LIVINGSTONE

Edinburgh London New York Oxford Philadelphia St Louis Sydney Toronto 2005

ELSEVIER
CHURCHILL
LIVINGSTONE

First published 2005
Reprinted 2005

ISBN 0 443 06462 8

British Library Cataloguing in Publication Data
A catalogue record for this book is available from the British Library

Library of Congress Cataloguing in Publication Data
A catalogue record for this book is available from the Library of Congress

Notice
Medical knowledge is constantly changing. Standard safety precautions must be followed, but as new research and clinical experience broaden our knowledge, changes in treatment and drug therapy may become necessary or appropriate. Readers are advised to check the most current product information provided by the manufacturer of each drug to be administered to verify the recommended dose, the method and duration of administration, and contraindications. It is the responsibility of the practitioner, relying on experience and knowledge of the patient, to determine dosages and the best treatment for each individual patient. Neither the Publisher nor the author assumes any liability for any injury and/or damage to persons or property arising from this publication.

The Publisher

ELSEVIER your source for books, journals and multimedia in the health sciences

www.elsevierhealth.com

Working together to grow
libraries in developing countries
www.elsevier.com | www.bookaid.org | www.sabre.org

 ELSEVIER BOOKAID International Sabre Foundation

The publisher's policy is to use paper manufactured from sustainable forests

Images on cover: see pages 15, 68, 140 and 300
Printed in China

Contents

Preface

Since the many advances in the use of ultrasound in imaging, several textbooks have been written on obstetrics and gynaecology ultrasound. This book, as its name suggests, is a study guide to help the student and practising sonographer. The questions are those that test the reader's academic knowledge and application in the practical scenario. The questions, as much as it is possible, have been grouped into sections so that when used in conjunction with the available textbooks and current research findings, learning can be systematic and individually tailored. Most ultrasound departments have a protocol governing obstetrics and gynaecology practices; the student/sonographer is encouraged to become familiar with this.

Ultrasound plays an important role in the evaluation and treatment of infertility and many sonographers are now finding that they are involved in this aspect of medicine. A chapter has been included in this book to introduce the sonographer to this rapidly advancing area of gynaecology and help the sonographer practising in this field.

The questions have been drawn from the lecture notes, journals, textbooks and practical experience of the author and many other colleagues.

London 2005   Oluwakemi O. Ola-Ojo

Acknowledgements

Many people and companies have been of great help to me in the writing of this book either by way of support, advice or permission to use some of their images or use extracts from their published work.

I am particularly grateful to: Professor K. Nicolaides, Mr O. E. Ojo, Dr S. Bower, Dr L. Gertz, Dr Massouh, Dr James Wafula, Mr Sam Abdalla and Miss Mary Power. Many thanks to my colleagues including Mrs J. Hollingsworth and her team of sonographers, Miss P. Wilson and her team of sonographers, Mr Z. M. Ahmed, and many other colleagues who would prefer to be anonymous.

My thanks to the following NHS Trust institutions from whom the images for the book were obtained: Frimley Park Hospital, Harris Birthright Research Centre for Fetal Medicine, St Thomas' Hospital, The County Hospital, The Lister Hospital – Assisted Conception Unit, Queen Charlotte, Hammersmith and Chelsea Hospitals and Queen Elizabeth Hospital.

Thanks to the following companies for giving me permission to reproduce the following images of their ultrasound equipment: Shimadzu Corporation for Fig. 2.40a; Aloka Co. Ltd for Fig. 2.40b; Hitachi Medical Corporation for Figs 2.40c and 2.40d. Thanks to Reed Business Information, Macmillan Publishers, Harper Collins Publishers. Thanks to the British Medical Ultrasound Society for the use of the obstetrics charts (adapted from BMUS Bulletin November 1994) and to Churchill Livingstone for the use of the 2nd trimester obstetric dating charts (adapted) in the appendix.

Many thanks to Mr Olanrewaju for sorting out my computer problems, and to Mr Andy Richardson and his team of librarians.

My profound gratitude to my friends and family for their patience and understanding all these years.

Thanks to my publishers, especially Mrs Mary Law, Mrs Sarena Wolfaard, Mrs Dinah Thom and Mrs Joannah Duncan, to the various reviewers and to Mrs Black the Copy Editor.

Finally I am grateful to Lady Eniola Olubobokun without whom the project could not have taken off and Mr O. Josiah without whose help the project could not have been concluded.

Glossary of abbreviations

4C	four chamber
a/40	a = gestational age; /40 = average length of a normal pregnancy
A&E	Accident and Emergency Department
Aao	ascending aorta
ABDC	amniotic band disruption complex
ABS	amniotic band syndrome
AC	abdominal circumference
AFI	amniotic fluid index
AFP	alphafetoprotein
AID	artificial insemination by donor
AIH	artificial insemination by husband
AIUM	American Institute of Ultrasound in Medicine
ANC	antenatal clinic
Ao	aorta
AP	anteroposterior
APD	anteroposterior diameter
APH	antepartum haemorrhage
ASD	atrial septal defect
ASGA	asymmetrical small for gestational age
AVHR	anterior ventricular hemisphere ratio
AVSD	atrioventricular septal defect
b/52	b = number of weeks; /52 = number of weeks in a year
BMUS	British Medical Ultrasound Society
BPD	biparietal diameter
bpm	beats per minute
c + d/40	c = gestational age in weeks; + d = days;
CAM	cystic adenomatoid malformation
CFD	colour-flow Doppler
CHD	congenital heart disease
ci	cephalic index
CLC	corpus luteal cyst
CM	cisterna magna
CMV	cytomegalovirus
CNS	central nervous system
COC	combined oral contraceptive
CPC	choroid plexus cyst

CRL	crown–rump length
CSF	cerebrospinal fluid
CT	computed tomography
CVS	chorionic villi sampling
CWD	continuous wave Doppler
D&C	dilation and curettage
DA	diamniotic
Dao	descending aorta
DC	dichorionic
DS	dating scan
DVT	deep vein thromobosis
DZ	dizygotic
EDD	expected date of delivery
EDF	end diastolic frequency
EFSUMB	European Federation of Societies for Ultrasound in Medicine and Biology
EGA	estimated gestational age
EPU	Early Pregnancy Unit
ERCP	evacuation of retained products of conception
ET	embryo transfer
FBM	fetal breathing movements
FET	frozen embryo transfer
FHB	fetal heartbeat
FL	femur length
FMU	Fetal Medicine Unit
FO	foramen ovale
FSH	follicle stimulating hormone
GA	gestational age
GIFT	gamete intrafallopian transfer
GIT	gastrointestinal tract
GP	general practitioner
GS	gestational sac
GSD	gestational sac diameter
GSV	gestational sac volume
GTT	glucose tolerance test
HBP	high blood pressure
HBSS	haemoglobin SS (sickle cell disease)
HC	head circumference
hCG	human chorionic gonadotrophin
HFEA	Human Fertilisation and Embryology Authority
HIS	hospital information system
HIV	human immunodeficiency virus
HSG	hysterosalpingogram, hysterosalpingography
IAS	interatrial septum
ICPC	isolated choroid plexus cyst

ICSI	intracytoplasmic sperm injection
IMB	intramenstrual bleeding in a year
IUCD	intrauterine contraceptive device
IUD	intrauterine death
IUGR	intrauterine growth retardation
IUGS	intrauterine gestational sac
IV	intravenous
IVC	inferior vena cava
IVF	in vitro fertilization
IVS	interventricular septum
KC	kidney circumference
LA	left atrium; local anaesthetic
LFT	liver function test
LH	luteinizing hormone
LH-RH	luteinizing hormone-releasing hormone
LIF	left iliac fossa
LMP	last menstrual period
LS	longitudinal section
LUF	luteinized unruptured follicle
LV	left ventricle; liquor volume
LVOT	left ventricular outflow tract
MA	monoamniotic
MAPD	maximum amniotic fluid pool vertical diameter
MB	moderator band
MC	monochorionic
MCA	middle cerebral artery
MCO	multicystic ovary
MKD	multicystic kidney disease
MoM	multiples of the median
MOT	malignant ovarian teratoma
MRI	magnetic resonance imaging
MSAFP	maternal serum alphafetoprotein
MV	mitral valve
MZ	monozygotic
NF	nuchal fold
NHS	National Health Service
NT	nuchal thickness
NTD	neural tube defect
OA	occipitoanterior
OCP	oral contraceptive pill
OFD	occipitofrontal diameter
OHSS	ovarian hyperstimulation syndrome
OP	occipitoposterior
PA	pulmonary artery

PACS	picture archiving and communication systems
PAPP	Papanicolaou test (exfoliative cell smear test)
PCO	polycystic ovary
PCOD	polycystic ovarian disease
PD	pulsed Doppler
PDA	patent ductus arteriosus
PI	pulsatility index
PID	pelvic inflammatory disease
PM	postmortem
PMB	postmenopausal bleeding
POD	pouch of Douglas
PPH	postpartum haemorrhage
PROM	premature rupture of the membranes
PS	postscript
PUJO	pelviureteric junction obstruction
PV	per vagina; pulmonary vein
PVHR	posterior ventricular hemisphere ratio
RA	right atrium
RI	resistance index
RIF	right iliac fossa
RPOC	retained products of conception
RV	right ventricle
RVOT	right ventricular outflow tract
S/D ratio	systolic/diastolic ratio
SAR	scatter, absorption, reflection
SD	standard deviation
SFD	small for dates
SGA	small for gestational age
SLE	systemic lupus erythematosus
SROM	spontaneous rupture of the membranes
SSGA	symmetrical small for gestational age
STD	sexually transmitted disease
SUZI	subzonal insemination
TA	transabdominal
TAS	transabdominal scan
TCD	transcerebellar diameter
TD	transverse diameter
TGC	time gain compensation
TLC	tender loving care
TOP	termination of pregnancy
TORCH	**t**oxoplasmosis, **o**ther infections, **r**ubella, **c**ytomegalovirus, **h**erpes simplex virus
TRAP	twin reversed arterial perfusion sequence
TS	transverse section
TTTS	twin–twin transfusion syndrome

TV	transvaginal; tricuspid valve
TVS	transvaginal scan
UB	urinary bladder
Ue	oestriol
UKAS	United Kingdom Association of Sonographers
US	ultrasound
VSD	ventricular septal defect
WFUMB	World Federation of Ultrasound in Medicine and Biology
WHO	World Health Organization
YS	yolk sac
ZIFT	zygote intrafallopian transfer

Symbols

–ve	negative
+ve	positive
<	less than
≤	less than or equal to
≥	equal to or more than

SECTION 1

Questions

SECTION CONTENTS

Anatomy

LEARNING OBJECTIVES

By the end of working through this chapter the reader should:

- know the anatomy and the functions of the ovaries, uterus and uterine tubes
- recognize the ultrasound pattern of normal ovarian and uterine anatomy
- recognize the ultrasound pattern of the normal 1st, 2nd and 3rd trimester fetal anatomy
- understand the menstrual cycle
- recognize the ultrasound pattern and the functions of a normal placenta
- understand the anatomy of the umbilical cord
- understand congenital anomalies and some of their causes.

INTRODUCTION

In order to be able to identify abnormal ultrasound appearances, a good knowledge of the normal and possible variants is necessary. For the sonographer, pattern recognition and understanding the possible causes of an abnormal ultrasound appearance and what such may imply will enhance professional practice. Unlike in some other diagnostic imaging techniques where the planes and the methods for obtaining the planes are fixed, in ultrasound examination, flexibility of the sonographer's technique is required to obtain the necessary views. Other challenges during any obstetric scan may include a moving fetus, unfavourable fetal position, maternal adipose tissue, poly- or oligohydramnios. In gynaecology ultrasound, one of the greatest challenges for the sonographer is the ability to link a particular ultrasound appearance to the possible pathology. Hands-on experience provides a good route to ultrasound pattern recognition.

In the UK, it is estimated that about 70% of those who perform obstetrics ultrasound are primarily radiographers; however, throughout this book, the term sonographer is used for the person who performs the ultrasound examination irrespective of their professional background or gender.

QUESTIONS

1 a] Describe the anatomy of the uterus.
   b] Describe the common anomalies of the uterus.
2 List the main functions of the uterus.
3 Describe the relationship of the uterus to the other pelvic organs.
4 What are the following?:
   — internal os
   — external os
   — endometrium
   — myometrium
   — perimetrium.
5 Describe the anatomy of the ovary.
6 a] What is the anatomical position of the ovary?
   b] What factors may affect the location of the ovaries?
   c] What factors can affect the size of the ovary?
7 What are the main functions of the ovary?

1.10a

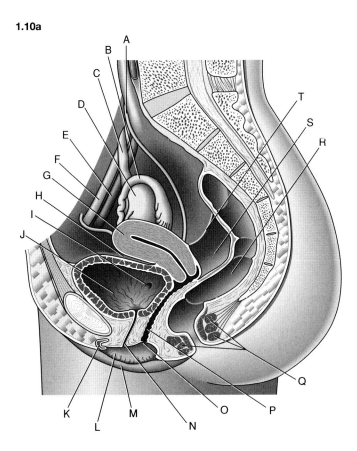

1.10b

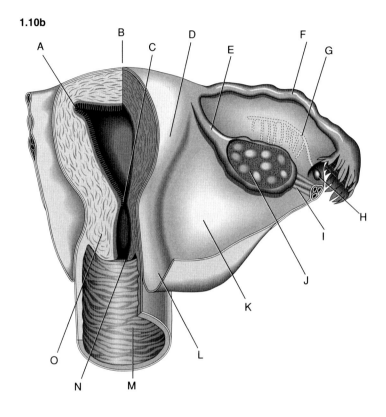

1.10c

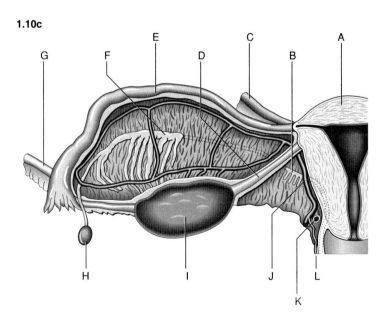

8 a] Describe the anatomy of the uterine tubes.
   b] What is the function of the uterine tubes?
   c] Describe the infundibulum of the uterine tube.
   d] Describe the ampulla of the uterine tube.
   e] Describe the isthmus of the uterine tube.
   f] What is a blocked tube and what causes this?
   g] What is the clinical significance of a blocked tube?
9 a] How can you recognize the vagina on the transabdominal (TA) scan?
   b] What is haematocolpos?
   c] What are the anterior, lateral and posterior fornices?
10 Identify the structures in Fig. 1.10a–c.
11 a] Identify the structures in Fig. 1.11a–g.
   b] Identify the types of section in Fig. 1.11a–g.

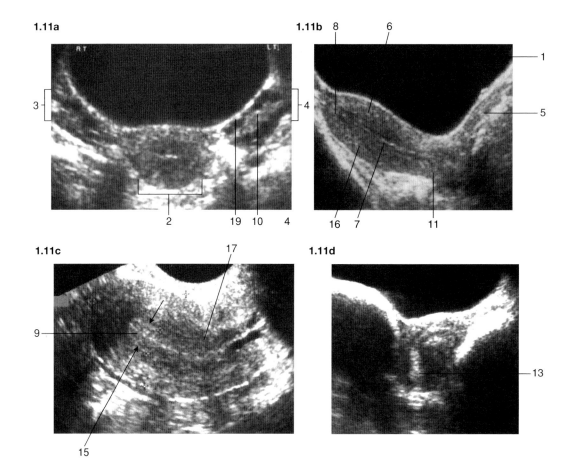

1.11a

1.11b

1.11c

1.11d

1.11e

1.11f

1.11g

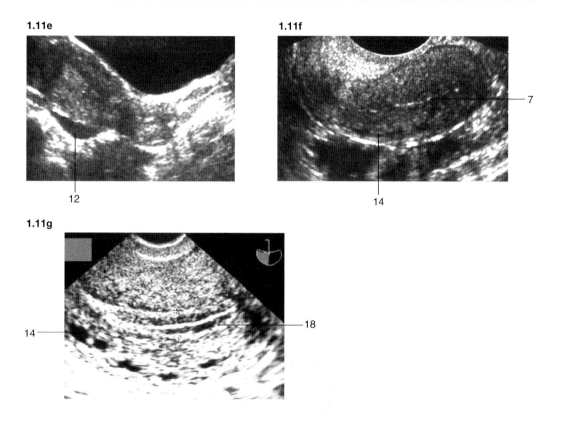

c] What is the difference between the structures labelled 7, 9, 13 and 18 and with which phase of the menstrual cycle could they be associated?

d] What is the difference between Fig. 1.11b and c, and Fig. 1.11b and d?

12 a] Which diagnostic imaging techniques could be used to assess the non-pregnant uterus, uterine tube and ovaries?

b] What are the advantages and disadvantages of these imaging techniques?

13 Describe the menstrual cycle.

14 a] Why is the POD a common site for fluid collection?

b] When is fluid seen in the POD?

15 Where is the oocyte usually fertilized by a sperm?

16 Immediately following fertilization, what is the fertilized ovum called?

17 What is the name for the fertilized ovum by the time it descends into the uterus?

18 a] When is the yolk sac seen on ultrasound?

b] Of what significance is the yolk sac?

19 What is the vitelline duct?

20 a] Identify the structures in Fig. 1.20a–k.

b] Approximately how old is the fetus in Fig. 1.20d?

c] What is being measured between + and + in Fig. 1.20e?

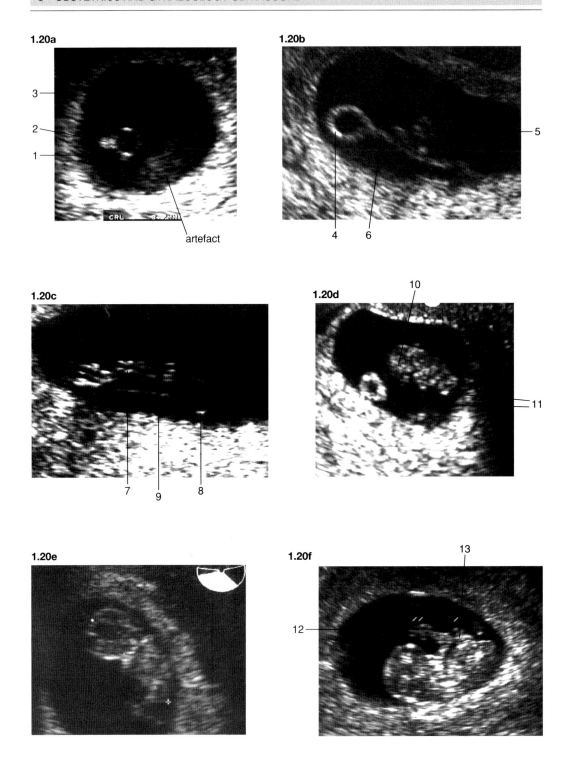

1.20a

3
2
1
artefact

1.20b

5
4 6

1.20c

7 9 8

1.20d

10
11

1.20e

1.20f

13
12

1.20g

14

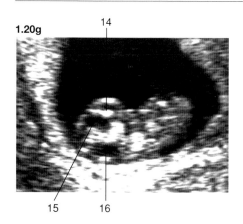

15 16

1.20h

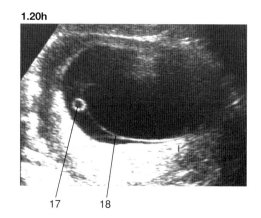

17 18

1.20i

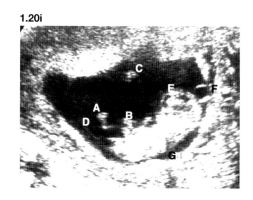

C
F F
A
D B
G

1.20j

19 25

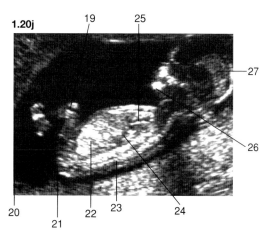

27

26

20 21 22 23 24

1.20k

33 32 31 30 28

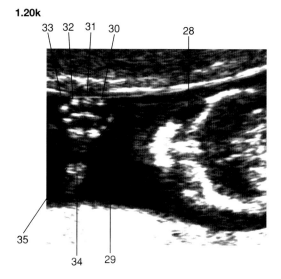

35
34 29

21 What is the difference between the embryonic and the fetal period?

22 a] What are chromosomes?

 b] What is a gene?

 c] How does the gene affect the individual make up?

 d] Which factors could lead to genetic abnormality?

 e] What are karyotypes?

23 What are the following?

 — chromosomal abnormality

 — congenital abnormality

 — genetic abnormality

 — anomaly

 — malformation.

24 What are some of the causes of congenital abnormalities?

25 a] What is congenital deformation?

 b] List some types of congenital deformation.

 c] What are the causes of congenital deformation?

26 What is a syndrome?

27 In which ways may a birth defect present?

28 What is a dysplasia?

29 a] What is an aneuploidy?

 b] What is polyploidy?

30 Why do Down's syndrome individuals look alike more than their own siblings?

31 How do environmental factors such as drugs cause congenital anomalies?

32 Which maternal illnesses can be associated with an increased risk of fetal malformation?

33 What is a teratogen?

34 Does the maternal blood normally intermingle with the fetal blood?

35 What is the clinical significance of intermingling of the fetal blood with the maternal blood (e.g. during an invasive procedure)?

36 What is the role of the placenta in the uteroplacental circulation?

37 Describe the functions of the placenta.

38 Describe the transport mechanism of the placenta.

39 Which substances may pass from the mother to the fetus and from the fetus to the mother via the placenta?

40 Identify which of the following is transferable or not transferable through the placental membrane: bacteria, oxygen, water, carbohydrate, lipids, amino acid, drugs, poison, heparin, viruses (e.g. rubella, CMV), radioactive substances such as strontium 90, antibodies, carbon monoxide, IgS and IgM, IgG and vitamins.

41 Why is heparin not transferable in the uteroplacental circulation?

42 What causes placental insufficiency?

43 What is the effect of the retention of an accessory placenta post-delivery?

44 How does nicotine in cigarette smoke affect uteroplacental circulation?

45 What is the function of human chorionic gonadotrophin (hCG) in early pregnancy?

46 Describe:
  a] the anatomy of the umbilical cord.
  b] the function of the umbilical cord.
  c] the causes of twisting of the umbilical cord.
47 a] What is included in a two-vessel umbilical cord?
  b] What causes it?
  c] What is its significance?
48 When is the matured external genitalia established in utero?
49 When does urine formation begin in utero?
50 What makes up the amniotic fluid?
51 a] What are the functions of the amniotic fluid?
  b] What are the possible effects/significance of premature rupture of the
     membranes (PROM) in pregnancy?

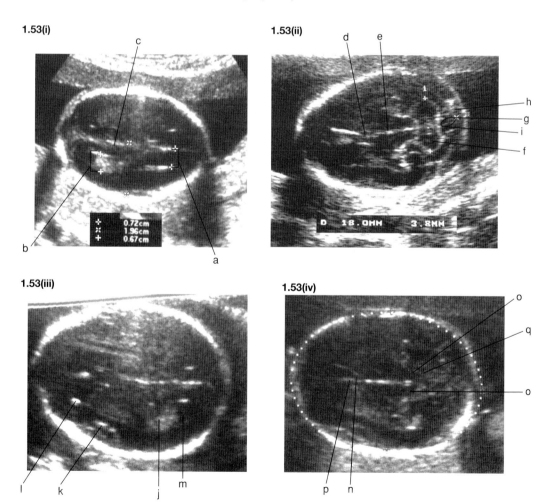

1.53(i)

1.53(ii)

1.53(iii)

1.53(iv)

1.53(v)

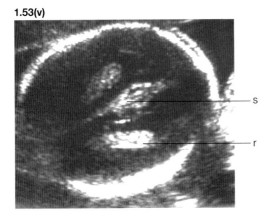

52 In what way is the amniotic fluid similar to the fluid in the fetus?
53 a] Identify the structures in Fig. 1.53i–v.
   b] Identify the sections and indicate what each demonstrates.
   c] What is being measured in Fig. 1.53i and 1.53ii and what is their clinical significance?
54 a] Identify the structures in Fig. 1.54a–n.
   b] Identify the sections and indicate what each demonstrates.
   c] What is the difference between Fig. 1.54f and 1.54n?
55 a] Identify the structures in Fig. 1.55i–viii.
   b] Identify the sections and indicate what each demonstrates.
56 What causes most congenital anomalies of the spinal cord?
57 What does spina bifida mean?
58 a] When are the limbs formed?
   b] What causes limb deformation?
   c] What is the incidence of limb malformation?
   d] Identify the structures in Fig. 1.58a–f.

1.54a   **1.54b**

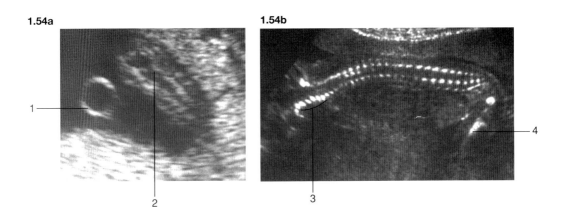

1.54c

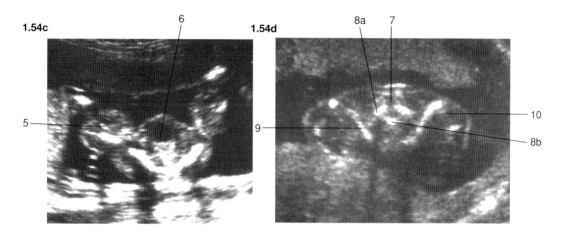

1.54e

1.54f

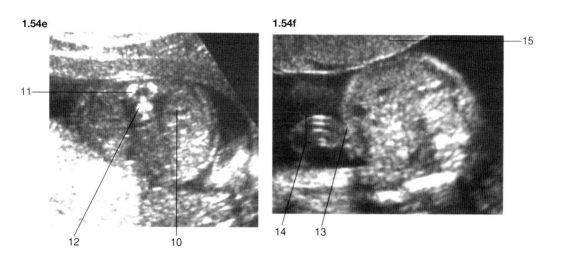

1.54g

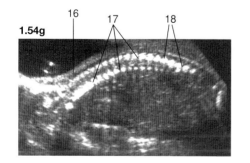

1.54h

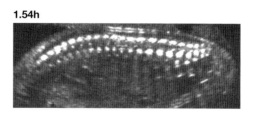

1.54i

1.54j

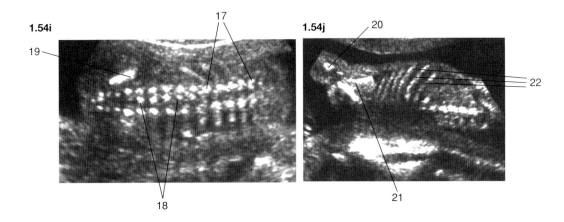

1.54k

1.54l

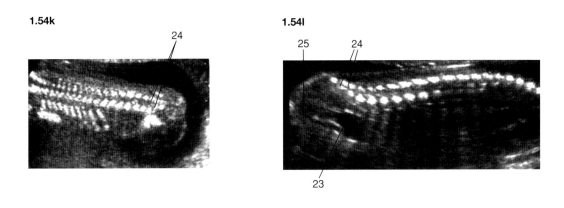

1.54m

1.54n

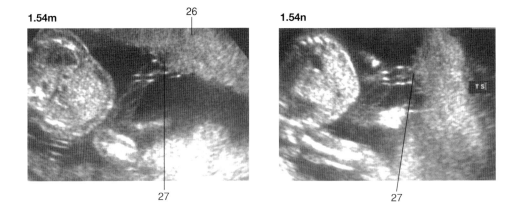

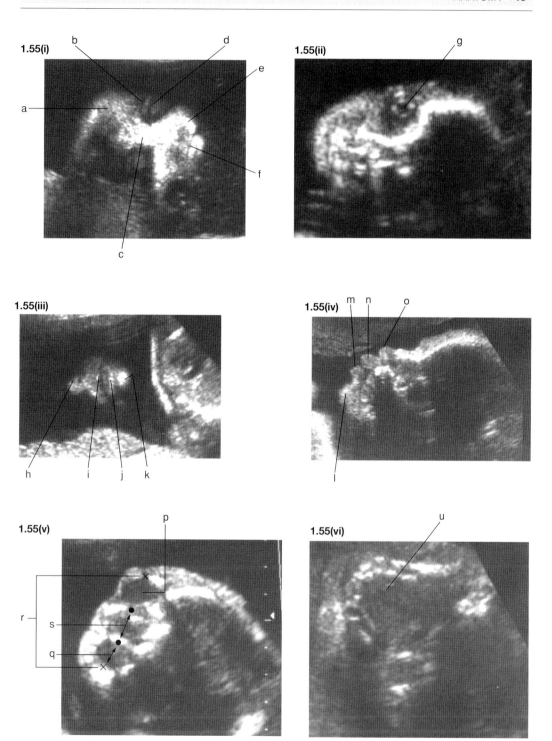

1.55(i)

a b c d e f

1.55(ii)

g

1.55(iii)

h i j k

1.55(iv)

l m n o

1.55(v)

p q r s

1.55(vi)

u

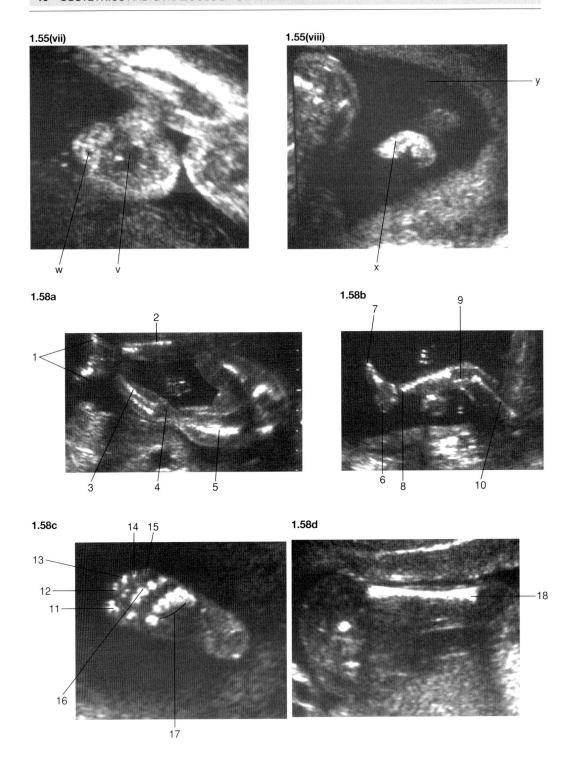

1.55(vii)

w   v

1.55(viii)

y

x

1.58a

2

1

3   4   5

1.58b

7   9

6   8   10

1.58c

14 15

13

12

11

16

17

1.58d

18

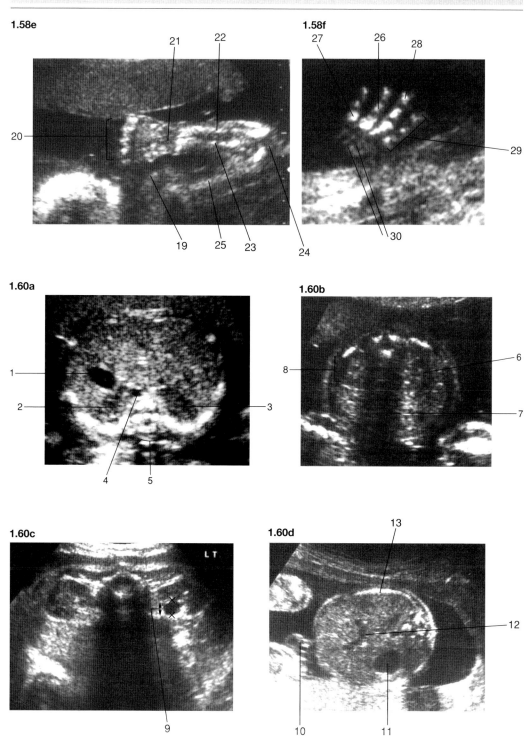

1.58e

1.58f

1.60a

1.60b

1.60c

1.60d

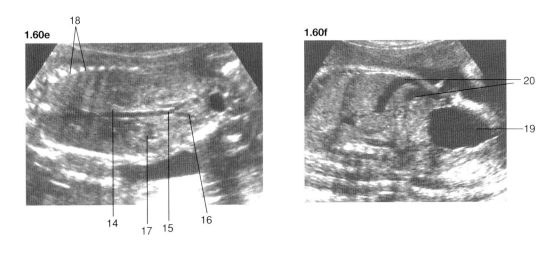

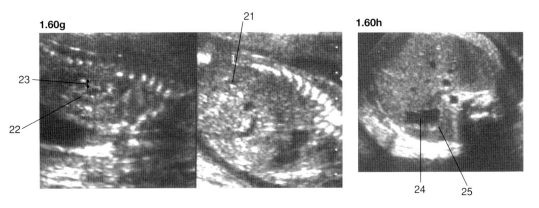

59 a] Which imaging techniques may be used to assess the fetus, especially when planning fetal treatment?

b] What are the advantages and disadvantages of such techniques compared with ultrasound?

60 Identify the structures in Fig. 1.60a–h.

61 a] Identify the structures in Fig. 1.61a–c.

b] Identify the sections in Fig. 1.61a–c.

62 a] What is TORCH?

b] How can TORCH affect the fetus?

63 a] What is VATER syndrome?

b] Which fetal structures should the sonographer check when the above syndrome is suspected?

1.61a

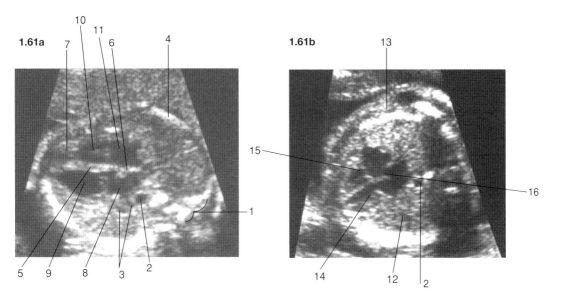

1.61b

1.61c

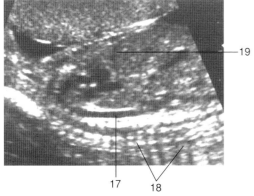

64 Identify the structures in Fig. 1.64a–c (images aimed at identifying fetal sex).

65 a] Identify the structures in Fig. 1.65a, b.

 b] Identify the sections in Fig. 1.65a, b.

 c] i] How was the lady in Fig. 1.65c scanned?

  ii] Identify a–d in Fig. 1.65c.

  iii] What is being measured between + and +?

1.64a

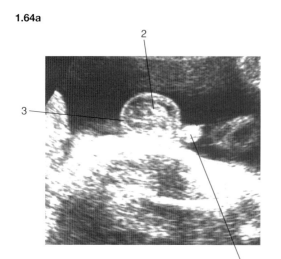

1.64b

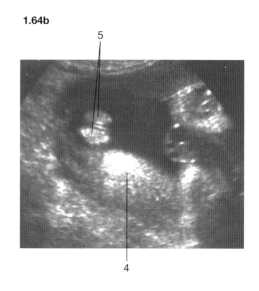

1.64c

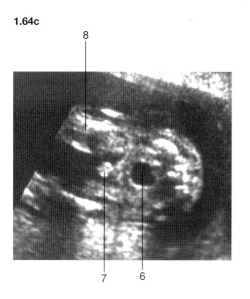

1.65a

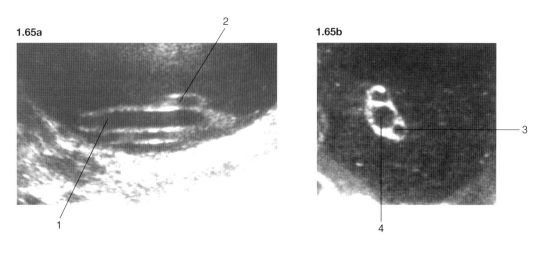

1.65b

1.65c

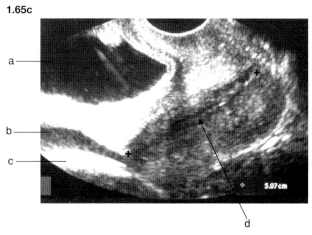

Q.2

Physics and instrumentation

LEARNING OBJECTIVES

By the end of working through this chapter the reader should:

- understand what ultrasound is and its safety
- understand ultrasound beam focusing
- understand ultrasound image resolution
- know the different types of transducer used in obstetrics and gynaecology
- understand the difference between static and real-time scanning
- understand the types and effects of artefacts and unsharpness
- be aware of quality assurance matters and ultrasound equipment maintenance
- know the various types of ultrasound image display, image storage facilities and hard copies
- understand Doppler and how it relates to obstetrics and gynaecology ultrasound.

INTRODUCTION

A knowledge of physics is essential to understanding how the equipment works, to operate the equipment appropriately and to identify artefacts and their effects on ultrasound images. Patients' awareness is now greater than in the past and questions relating to the safety of ultrasound in medical practice are not uncommon.

It has been suggested that lack of toxicity has allowed ultrasound to have an enviable record for safety such that 'more than one out of every four imaging studies in the world is an ultrasound study'.

Quality assurance of ultrasound equipment has become essential as perfect stability cannot be achieved even in modern ultrasound equipment. Some variation is to be expected and, in order to measure significant changes and to detect faults as quickly, regular monitoring is essential.

There are many ways of acquisition and storage of ultrasound images and the sonographer should be aware of what is available and be able to operate these systems. The sonographer should also be aware of their organization's protocol governing image acquisition and its storage.

Sonographers – as one of the prime users of the ultrasound equipment – are becoming more involved in the purchase of such equipment and therefore have to be aware of what is available and keep up-to-date with the changes in technology in order to enhance professional practice.

3D imaging in obstetrics and gynaecology appears very promising but its routine use by sonographers in a typical district general hospital is unclear at present.

The questions in this chapter have been tailored to what is currently applicable to routine sonography practice.

◆ Protocols may vary from one unit to another.

QUESTIONS

1 How would you explain to Lady A (a patient):
  a] What ultrasound is?
  b] How ultrasound is produced?
  c] Why the coupling gel is used in/for ultrasound examinations?
  d] Why is it important to use the manufacturer's recommended coupling gel?
2 a] What is the difference between noise and sound?
  b] What are the following?:
   • amplitude of a waveform
   • wavelength
   • frequency.
3 What is the piezoelectric effect?
4 What determines the frequency of ultrasound produced by a piezoelectric element?
5 What is the resonant frequency?
6 How is a piezoelectric material such as zirconate titanate able to transmit and receive current?
7 What is the velocity of ultrasound in most soft tissue?

Ultrasound beam/focusing

8 What is the difference in the beam direction between transabdominal (TA) and transvaginal scan (TVS)?
9 List the processes by which the intensity of transmitted ultrasound is decreased.
10 Describe how these processes achieve their effect.
11 What is the clinical significance of scatter, reflection and absorption (SAR)?
12 What is refraction?
13 Why is it important to keep the beam perpendicular to the interface if possible?
14 a] What is the focal length?
  b] What is the difference between the Fresnel zone and the Fraunhofer zone?
  c] Identify a–g in Fig. 2.14.
15 a] What is beam/transducer focusing?
  b] How can focusing of the ultrasound beam be achieved?
16 How is electronic focusing achieved?

2.14

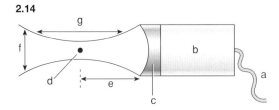

Image resolution

17 What is resolution?
18 What is the difference between axial and lateral resolution?

Transducers

19 List and describe the various types of conventional transducer head.
20 List some specialized transducers.
21 Which factors may determine the choice of transducer for an ultrasound examination?
22 What are some of the limitations of using a contact compound scanner?
23 What is a phased array scanner?
24 Which ultrasound examination favours the use of the phased array scanner?
25 What is an interface?
26 What is a specular reflector?
27 List and describe the components of the transducer.

Static/real-time scanning/artefacts/unsharpness

28 What is the difference between real-time and static scan?
29 List the possible artefacts on real-time ultrasound scanning.
30 For each artefact above, describe the cause, the ultrasound (US) appearance and how it can be eliminated.
31 What are some of the effects of artefacts?
32 List some of the causes of unsharp ultrasound images.

Equipment quality assurance and maintenance

33 Describe quality assurance (QA) as it relates to ultrasound equipment.
34 Why is it important to perform QA tests on ultrasound equipment?
35 List the possible QA tests that can be performed on real-time ultrasound equipment and by whom.
36 In setting up a QA programme for the ultrasound department, what points should the sonographer bear in mind?
37 List the possible QA test that could be performed on the ultrasound equipment by the sonographer on a daily basis, a weekly basis, and a monthly basis.

38 What are some of the advantages of an ultrasound unit having its own test object rather than borrowing one from another hospital?

39 Describe how you would sterilize the transvaginal probe.

Equipment design and purchase

40 Fig. 2.40a shows an example of a portable digital colour Doppler ultrasound system, to which a video recorder can be added. Fig. 2.40b illustrates a detailed view of an example of a multipurpose operating platform.

2.40a

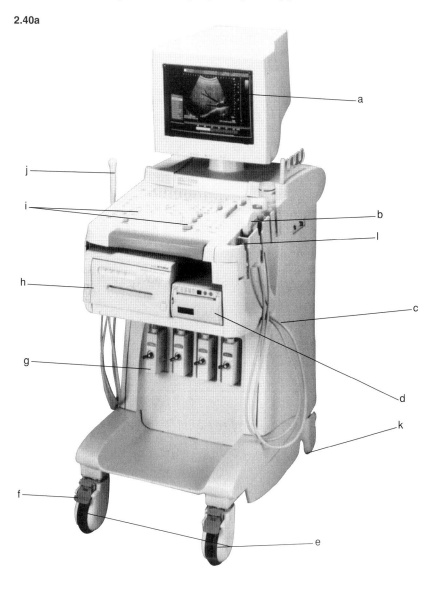

2.40b

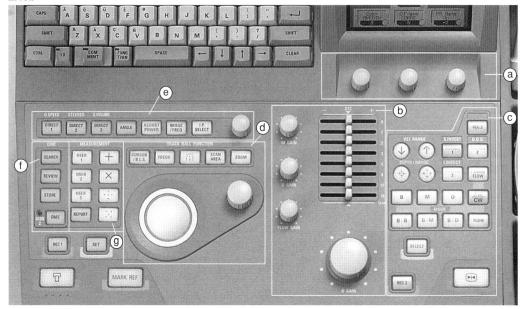

2.40c

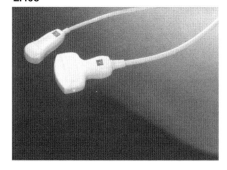

2.40d

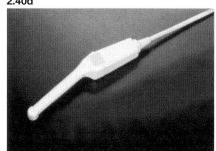

a] Identify a–l in Fig. 2.40a.

b] In Fig. 2.40b identify panels a-g.

c] Identify the probes illustrated in Fig. 2.40c and 2.40d.

d] How is 2-dimensional (2D) ultrasound different from volume mode ultrasonography?

e] In which way is 3-dimensional (3D) ultrasound equipment different from 2D ultrasound equipment?

f] In acquiring a 3-dimensional ultrasound image, which other specific controls on the ultrasound equipment will the sonographer select?

41 a] Describe the functions attributable to panels a-g in Fig. 2.40b.

b] Tissue harmonic echo, DMS, STC and DICOM are relatively new terms in ultrasonography. What do they describe?

42 List the possible factors that can influence the purchase of ultrasound equipment.

43 Your department in a district general hospital is about to provide an 'early pregnancy ultrasound service'.
  a] What factors would you consider in establishing this service?
  b] What sort of ultrasound equipment would you consider appropriate for this service?

Ultrasound safety

44 How safe is it to perform ultrasound of the first trimester embryo?

45 What precautions can be taken to ensure that a patient dose for an ultrasound scan is kept to a minimum?

46 List the broad range of ultrasound intensities currently available in the different diagnostic modalities and discuss the range for which higher intensities are required.

47 In which ways can the safety of modern ultrasound equipment be achieved/ensured?

48 a] Discuss the safety parameters necessary in ultrasound.
  b] Describe the thermal and non-thermal ultrasound bioeffects.
  c] What are the following:
    1. TI
    2. MI
    3. TIS
    4. TIB
    5. TIC
    6. (I_{SPTA})
    7. I_{SP}.

Image display, storage and hardcopy

49 What is the dynamic range?

50 List and describe the possible ways of displaying ultrasound images.

51 What causes image flickering?

52 List the possible methods of storing ultrasound images.

53 What are the advantages and disadvantages of each of these storage methods?

54 What is the difference between a multi-image and a multiformat camera?

55 Explain how the production of an ultrasound image differs from the production of a radiographic image.

56 In what way does the 'film' used for recording an ultrasound image differ from the type used for recording a conventional radiographic image?

Doppler

57 What is the Doppler principle?

58 How is depth calculated in ultrasound?

59 a] What is the difference between pulsed Doppler and continuous wave Doppler?
    b] What is the difference between colour-flow Doppler and power Doppler?
    c] What is aliasing?
60 Briefly describe how to obtain an umbilical artery Doppler waveform.
61 Which Doppler information can be suggestive of high vascular resistance within the placenta?
62 In which clinical conditions can this be found?
63 What is the clinical significance of the reversal of end-diastolic flow?
64 What is the clinical significance of absent end-diastolic flow?
65 What precautions should the sonographer take while conducting a Doppler study on a multiple pregnancy?
66 What factors can inhibit obtaining an umbilical artery waveform?
67 Identify the artefacts and their possible causes in Fig. 2.67a–d.

2.67a TVS right iliac fossa.

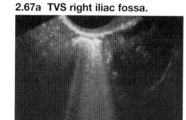

2.67b

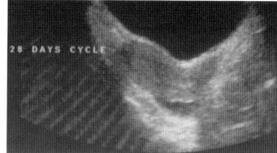

2.67c single fetus.

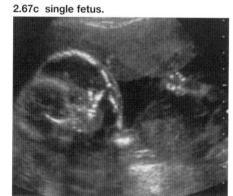

2.67d

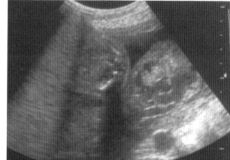

Gynaecology

LEARNING OBJECTIVES

By the end of working through this chapter the reader should:

- know how to prepare a patient for gynaecology scan and the various types of scanning approach
- be aware of the average adult uterine and ovarian measurements and the implications of measurements outside of this range
- be aware of some common gynaecological terminology
- know the various types of ultrasound appearance of the endometrium
- understand why gynaecology scan can be done for intrauterine contraceptive device (IUCD), the various types of IUCD, possible ultrasound appearances of IUCD, possible difficulties in identifying a missing IUCD, the information required following a scan for IUCD location and the possible risk with the use of IUCD
- understand what a leiomyoma is, why a gynaecology scan can be requested for leiomyoma, its possible location in the pelvis, techniques for scanning, difference between leiomyoma and Braxton Hicks and between leiomyoma and adenomyosis
- understand some common reasons for postmenopausal gynaecological scanning
- be aware of some endometrial/ovarian pathologies
- in each case presented be able to:
  - identify normal and abnormal ultrasound patterns in the images
  - write an ultrasound report from the images
  - suggest the possible condition/alternatives
  - suggest which organs/structures should be checked and why
  - understand the implications of the demonstrated conditions
  - be aware of the ultrasound role in the management of the case presented
  - be informed of the presented case outcome where known.

INTRODUCTION

The extensive use of ultrasound in the examination and assessment of the female pelvis may be attributed to many reasons. It is non-invasive, never contraindicated in any patient and not as expensive as some other diagnostic imaging modalities, usually available in most hospitals in the UK. However it is very operator dependent. Gynaecology ultrasound is usually requested to confirm the normality or otherwise of the female reproductive organs. It is important for the sonographer to be familiar with departmental protocol which should address all aspects of gynaecology scans, especially in relation to communicating the scan report and chaperoning, particularly for transvaginal scan.

QUESTIONS
General questions

1 Good communication with the patient is a very important part of a pelvic ultrasound examination. Why?

2 Why is it important to determine the source of a localized tenderness while scanning?

3 Which questions should the sonographer ask the patient before embarking on a gynaecology scan and why?

4 What is the difference between transabdominal (TA) scan and transvaginal scan (TVS) with regard to the scanning planes and the waves' transmission?

5 List the uses of ultrasound in the management of a pelvic mass.

Patient preparation/techniques

6 List at least eight clinical indications for transvaginal ultrasound (TVS).

7 List the possible contraindications to TVS.

8 For which pelvic conditions can TVS provide information additional to that from a TA scan of the pelvis?

9 What preparations are necessary before a TVS?

10 What are the limitations of a TVS?

11 When is TA superior to TVS in pelvic ultrasound examination?

12 A retroverted uterus is difficult to assess by the TA scan approach with or without a full bladder. Why?

13 What are some of the advantages of the patient having a full urinary bladder for a TA scan?

14 List the movements possible with a TV and a TA probe.

15 a] List the advantages of a TV scan over a TA scan in gynaecology and 1st trimester scan.
   b] List some gynaecological indications for a TV scan.
   c] List some indications for a TV scan in pregnancy.

Anatomy/measurements

16 a] What is the average uterus measurement in an adult?
   b] List some of the causes of an enlarged uterus.

17 Why is it sometimes difficult to delineate the lateral borders of the uterus when measuring the width?

18 a] How is the ovarian volume calculated?
   b] What is the average ovarian volume in an adult?
   c] What is the clinical significance of ovarian volume?
19 What is the significance of finding a genital tract anomaly?
20 What is a vaginal cuff?

Common gynaecological terminologies

21 a] What do the following terms mean?:
   — amenorrhoea
   — dysmenorrhoea
   — dyspareunia
   — oligomenorrhoea
   — menorrhagia
   — menometrorrhagia.
   b] In the above conditions, what is the role of ultrasound?
   c] What are: hydrometra, pyometra, hydrosalpinx and pyosalpinx?

Ultrasound appearances

22 How can hydrosalpinx be differentiated from ovarian cyst on ultrasound?
23 In which conditions can an increased amount of fluid be seen in the pouch of Douglas (POD) on ultrasound?
24 How can fresh blood clots be differentiated from old pelvic blood on ultrasound?
25 Which ultrasound findings can suggest pelvic adhesions?
26 Which clinical conditions should be suspected in a patient with ultrasound features of bilateral adnexal masses of varying echogenicity?
27 How can fluid- or stool-filled bowel loops be differentiated from a pelvic abscess on ultrasound?
28 How can pelvic ascites be differentiated from the urinary bladder on ultrasound?
29 In which clinical conditions could a woman of childbearing age have her uterus surgically removed but have her ovaries retained?
30 What is the advantage of performing a pelvic ultrasound over a pelvic examination in a patient with pelvic inflammatory disease (PID)?
31 List the uses of ultrasound in the evaluation of PID and postoperative collections.
32 What is the typical ultrasound appearance of a pyosalpinx?
33 What is the ultrasound difference in the appearance of pyosalpinx and hydrosalpinx?
34 What is the common ultrasound appearance of a pelvic abscess?
35 During a pelvic scan which points need to be noted with regard to the urinary bladder?
36 How does calcification of the arcuate artery present on ultrasound?
37 What is the clinical significance of a calcified arcuate artery?
38 Which ultrasound findings can be suggestive of uterine rupture in a patient following suction curettage?

39 For which gynaecological procedures can ultrasound be of use?

40 Describe the ultrasound appearances of the uterus and ovaries in a patient with Turner's syndrome.

41 Which pelvic ultrasound findings may suggest ovarian malignancy?

42 Which ultrasound features can suggest dermoid or cystic teratoma?

43 Upon the discovery of a pelvic mass on ultrasound what information should the sonographer document?

44 What is the typical ultrasound appearance of a simple ovarian cyst?

45 Which ultrasound appearances can suggest endometrioma (chocolate cyst)?

46 Which ultrasound features may suggest bicornuate uterus?

Endometriium

47 Describe the ultrasound-recognizable changes of the endometrium in a menstrual cycle.

48 Describe the ultrasound appearances of a normal menopausal endometrium.

49 In which way may an ultrasound scan be useful in endometrial assessment?

50 What is the significance of endometrial motion as seen during real-time scanning?

51 a] What is abnormal uterine bleeding?
    b] What causes it?
    c] What is the role of ultrasound in this condition?

52 Describe the ultrasound appearance of the endometrium which may be seen in patients on the combined oral contraceptive (COC) pill.

53 List some of the causes of a typical hyperechoic endometrium which measures ≥ 17 mm thick.

54 In which group of patients may the following ultrasound findings of the endometrium be seen? 'A typical poorly developed hyperechoic endometrium which is less hyperechoic and/or thinner than the usual luteal phase endometrium in spite of the central hyperechoic echo of the endometrial cavity.'

55 Where else should the sonographer check when a triple line or luteal phase endometrium is seen in a patient on oral contraceptive and why?

56 In which conditions could a mixed echo endometrium be seen?

57 In which conditions could a typically absent endometrium be seen?

58 In which conditions could a typically anechoic endometrium be seen?

59 In which conditions could a luteal phase endometrium be seen in a patient who is bleeding?

Contraceptive devices

60 For which patients is routine ultrasound scan recommended before an intrauterine contraceptive device (IUCD) is inserted?

61 List the possible clinical indications for an ultrasound scan of IUCD after insertion.

62 Following a scan for IUCD localization, what information should the sonographer document?

63 Where there is a coexisting pregnancy with an IUCD in situ, what information should the ultrasonographer document?

64 What is the clinical significance of a properly placed IUCD?

65 Where the IUCD cannot be located by ultrasound, which other diagnostic imaging techniques may be used to demonstrate the device?

66 Which ultrasound findings are suggestive of an embedded IUCD?

67 Which ultrasound findings can suggest:
    a] partial perforation by an IUCD
    b] complete perforation by an IUCD?

68 How best can a non-Mirena IUCD be confirmed in the uterus?

69 What else can mimic an IUCD in the uterus?

70 a] Recognition of an IUCD in a retroverted or retroflexed uterus can be a problem. Why?
    b] How can these problems be overcome?

71 a] How is the shape of Copper T differentiated from that of Copper 7 on ultrasound?
    b] Describe the ultrasound appearance of the Mirena coil on ultrasound.
    c] Why is the Mirena coil difficult to identify on ultrasound?
    d] Where a transabdominal scan (TAS) fails to demonstrate a missing Mirena coil, what else can the sonographer do?

72 List the possible risks with the use of an IUCD.

Leiomyoma

73 a] What is a leiomyoma?
    b] List and describe the possible locations of a leiomyoma and the significance of each position.
    c] Identify the location of the leiomyomas labelled a–g in Fig. 3.73c.

74 List the possible clinical indications for scanning a known leiomyoma.

75 Which ultrasound findings are suggestive of a leiomyoma?

76 How can Braxton Hicks be differentiated from leiomyoma on ultrasound?

3.73c

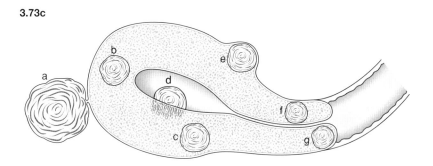

77 What is the difference between red degeneration of leiomyoma and hyaline degeneration?
78 Why may serial scans of the leiomyoma be requested in postmenopausal women?
79 It is sometimes better to scan a large leiomyoma using TAS rather than TVS. Why?
80 How does leiomyoma differ from adenomyosis on ultrasound?

Postmenopausal conditions

81 a] What is the clinical significance of postmenopausal bleeding?
   b] List some of the causes of postmenopausal bleeding.
82 Why are postmenopausal ovaries occasionally difficult to locate on ultrasound?
83 Which ultrasound findings of the ovaries of a postmenopausal patient can suggest ovarian problems?

Endometrial and ovarian pathology

84 a] What is a mucocele?
   b] How can a mucocele be differentiated from an ovarian dermoid?
85 Why would/could a woman of child-bearing age with a history of previous hysterectomy be referred for a pelvic scan?
86 What should the sonographer bear in mind when scanning the above patient and why?
87 What is a serous cystadenoma?
88 Which ultrasound findings can suggest serous cystadenoma?
89 How may serous cystadenocarcinoma present on ultrasound?
90 What are the possible complications of an ovarian mass?
91 a] What is the difference between endometriosis and adenomyosis?
   b] What is the difference in the clinical presentation of patients with endometriosis and patients with adenomyosis?
   c] What is endometritis?
   d] What causes endometritis?
   e] When the ultrasound result is positive for endometritis, which ultrasound features may be seen?
92 a] What is endometrial cancer?
   b] What are the symptoms of endometrial cancer?
   c] Which ultrasound findings can suggest endometrial cancer?
93 a] What is the incidence of benign ovarian teratoma?
   b] What is the use of ultrasound in the management of ovarian teratoma?
94 Which ultrasound findings can suggest cervical cancer?
95 List the possible ultrasound features that can suggest a malignant ovarian teratoma.

Case presentations

96 A teenager was referred for a scan with a history of lower abdominal pain, no PV bleed or discharge but with dyspareunia. Known 28-day regular cycle. Fig. 3.96 illustrates the ultrasound findings on day 19.
   a] Describe the ultrasound appearances.
   b] Is there is any possible ultrasound explanation for the pain?
   c] How is ultrasound useful in the management of this patient?
97 The image in Fig. 3.97 was taken during a diagnostic imaging examination.
   a] Which imaging procedure is this likely to be and what makes you think so?
   b] Which precautions need be considered when booking this investigation and why?
   c] What does Fig. 3.97 demonstrate?
98 This lady was referred for a scan with a history of a bulky uterus following delivery 25 days previously and tender and painful right iliac fossa (RIF). Fig. 3.98 shows the ultrasound findings. The left ovary was not identified.
   a] Describe the ultrasound appearances.
   b] Is there is any possible ultrasound-identifiable cause for the RIF pain?
   c] What is the use of ultrasound in the management of this patient?

3.96a

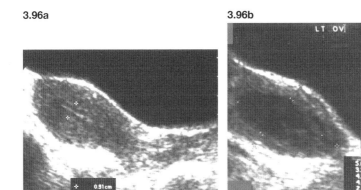

3.96b

3.96c

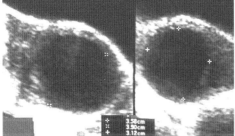

3.96d Right ovary measurement = 53 × 46 × 42 mm.

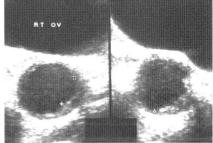

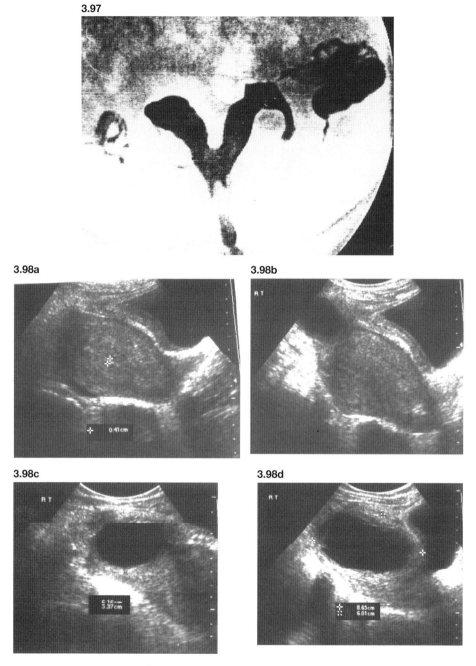

3.97

3.98a

3.98b

3.98c

3.98d

99 This lady in her fourth decade was referred with a history of continuous bleeding for a few months. Fig. 3.99 illustrates the ultrasound findings of the uterus.

3.99a

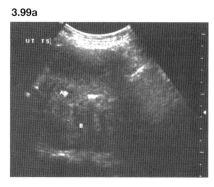

3.99b

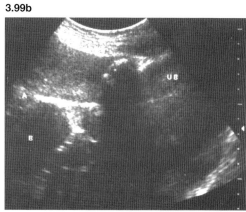

a] Describe the ultrasound appearances.
b] What is indicated by Fig. 3.99a and 3.99b?
c] What is the use of ultrasound in the management of this patient?
d] Which technical problems might be encountered by the sonographer in performing this ultrasound examination?

100 This lady in her forties was referred because of intramenstrual bleed. Fig. 3.100 demonstrates the ultrasound finding of the uterus.
a] Describe the ultrasound appearances.
b] What are the possible causes for intramenstrual bleeding in a patient with a negative pregnancy test result?
c] What is the aim of performing ultrasound in this lady?
d] Which other organ should be examined by the sonographer and why?

101 This lady in her twenties was referred with a history of RIF and primary infertility. The left ovary (not shown in Fig. 3.101) was $24 \times 20 \times 13$ mm and it appeared normal in outline and echopattern. The uterus was normal in outline, size and echopattern.

3.100a

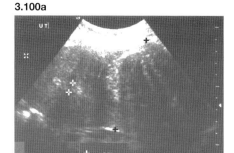

3.100b

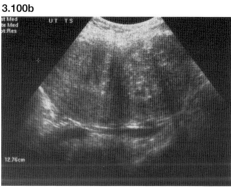

3.101a

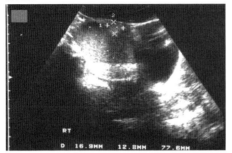

3.101b

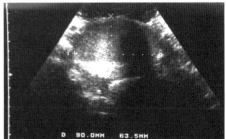

3.101c

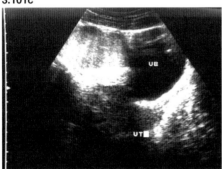

a] Describe the ultrasound appearances.

b] What is the possible condition demonstrated here and which other diagnostic imaging examination could help confirm this finding?

c] Is there any other possible anatomical cause for the RIF pain?

102 This lady in her late twenties was referred with a history of secondary amenorrhoea. Last menstrual period (LMP) was 182 days before the scan.

a] Calculate the ovarian volume.

b] Describe the ultrasound findings and identify the condition.

c] Which other non-invasive diagnostic test could be done to confirm or refute the ultrasound findings?

d] What could be responsible for this lady's long cycle?

e] What is the clinical significance of these findings?

103 This lady in her seventies was referred because of recent PV bleed. Menopause was 20 years before.

a] What is the role of ultrasound in the management of this lady?

b] Describe the ultrasound findings in Fig. 3.103.

104 This lady in her seventies was referred with a history of 1/52 PV bleed. She had never been on HRT. LMP about 20 years before. The left ovary (not shown in Fig. 3.104) was 21 × 19 × 14 mm. The right ovary was not identified.

a] Describe the ultrasound findings in Fig. 3.104.

b] Which conditions are demonstrated?

c] What might have been responsible for the PV bleed?

3.102a

3.102b

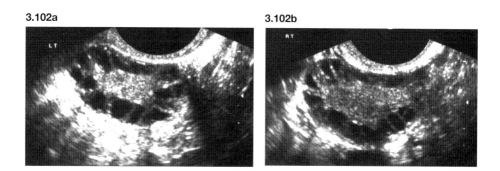

3.102c

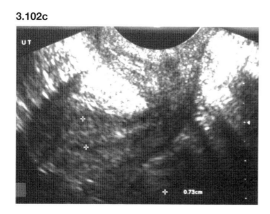

3.103a Uterus 47 × 38 × 37 mm.

3.103b

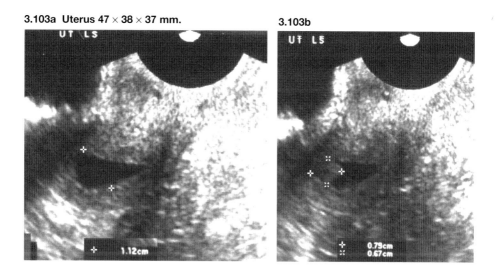

3.104a Uterus 93 × 65 × 65 mm.   **3.104b**

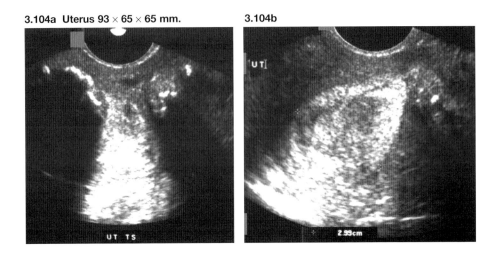

105 This lady in her thirties was referred with a history of continuous PV discharge. IUCD was fitted 10 years previously. Fig. 3.105 illustrates the ultrasound findings on day 20. She is known to have a 28–30-day cycle.
   a] Calculate the ovarian volume.
   b] Describe the ultrasound findings.
   c] In which way may ultrasound be used for further management of this lady?
106. This lady in her late twenties was referred with a history of primary infertility. LMP was 11/12 before the scan.
   a] Calculate the ovarian volume.
   b] Describe the ultrasound appearances.
   c] Which other non-invasive diagnostic tests may be requested by the clinician that can assist in the interpretation of the ultrasound findings?

3.105a   **3.105b**

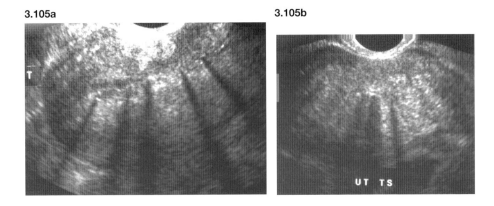

3.105c Right ovary measurement
= 78 × 71 × 61 mm.

3.105d

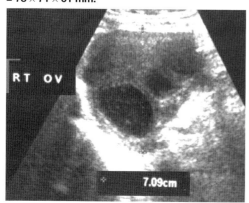

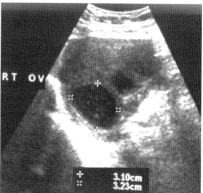

3.105e Left ovary measurement = 55 × 55 × 54 mm.

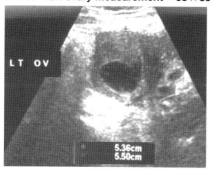

3.106a

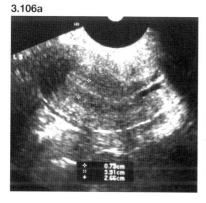

3.106b Left ovary 35 × 31 × 17 mm; right ovary
34 × 30 × 23 mm

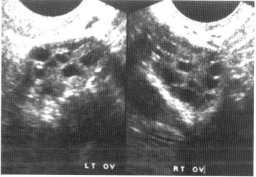

107 This 44-year-old lady was referred for a pelvic scan with a history of menorrhagia. Ultrasound findings on day 19 of a 28-day cycle are shown in Fig. 3.107. Both ovaries (not shown here) appeared normal in echopattern and size.

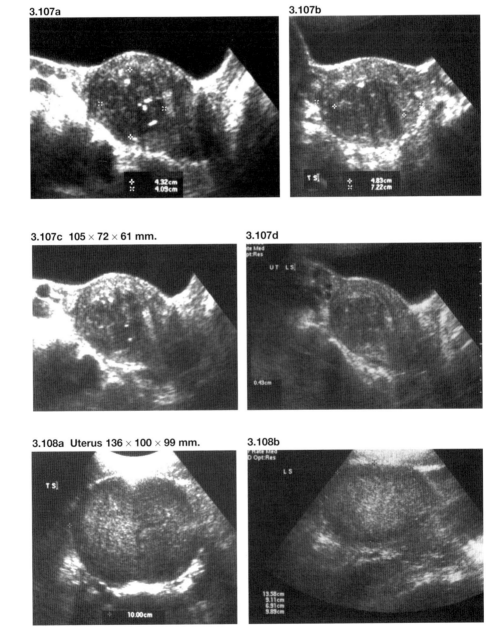

3.107a

3.107b

3.107c 105 × 72 × 61 mm.

3.107d

3.108a Uterus 136 × 100 × 99 mm.

3.108b

a] Describe the ultrasound appearances.

b] What may be the cause of this lady's menorrhagia?

108   This lady in her twenties was referred because of a possible mass in the midline and heavy menstrual periods. The ultrasound findings of the uterus are illustrated in Fig. 3.108.

a] Describe the ultrasound appearances.

b] What can this entity be?

109   This lady in her twenties was referred with a history of irregular bleeding. Both ovaries (not shown in Fig. 3.109) were normal in ultrasound appearance.

3.109a   **3.109b**

3.109c   **3.109d**

3.109e 0.99 mm.

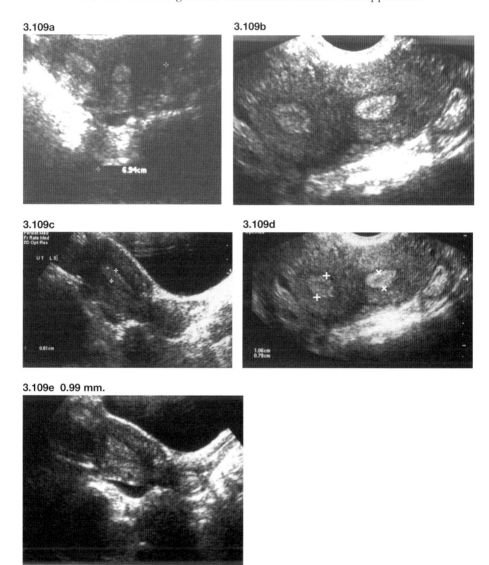

a] Describe the ultrasound appearances.
b] What is the likely condition?

110 This lady was referred for a scan with a history of pelvic pain but no history of previous abdominal surgery.
a] Identify the structures labelled a–c in Fig. 3.110.
b] Describe the ultrasound appearances as shown in Fig. 3.110a–b.
c] What do you notice about the body markers?
d] Is there any other significant finding in this lady?

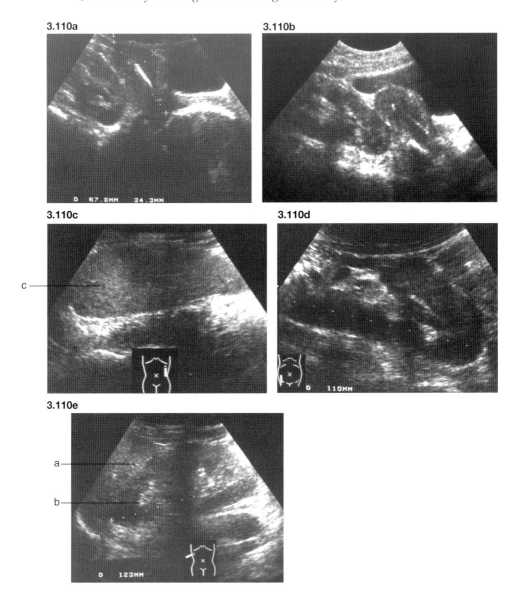

3.110a
3.110b
3.110c
3.110d
3.110e

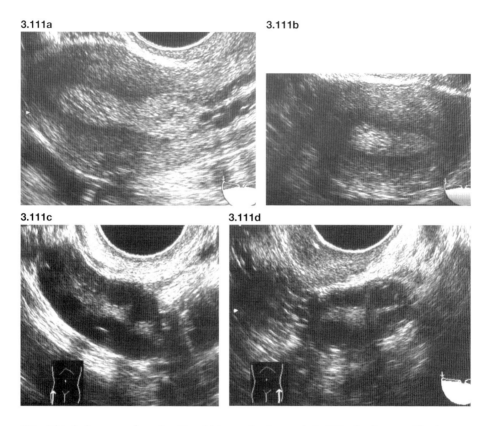

3.111a 3.111b
3.111c 3.111d

111   This lady was referred with a history of primary infertility for 3 years. She is
known to have up to two menstrual periods in a year. The ultrasound findings
are illustrated in Fig. 3.111.
a] Describe the ultrasound appearances.
b] What is the diagnosis?
c] What is the clinical significance of these findings?

112   Lady A in her seventies was referred for a pelvic scan to rule out ovarian
pathology. The ovaries were not identified.
Lady B, who was much younger, had a routine gynaecological scan.
Both ovaries (not shown here) were normal in outline and echopattern. Fig. 3.112
illustrates the other ultrasound findings in both ladies.
a] Describe the ultrasound appearances seen in Lady A and Lady B.
b] What are the likely diagnoses?
c] What is the clinical significance of these findings?

113   This lady was referred with a history of severe pelvic cramps and bleeding
following IUCD insertion. Both ovaries (not shown in Fig. 3.113) were of normal
appearance.
a] Describe the ultrasound appearances.
b] What is the clinical significance of this finding?

3.112a Lady A.

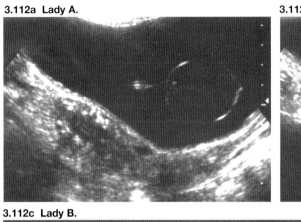

3.112b Transverse section.

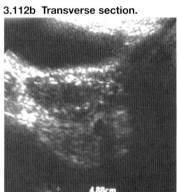

3.112c Lady B.

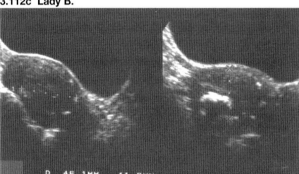

3.113a

3.113b

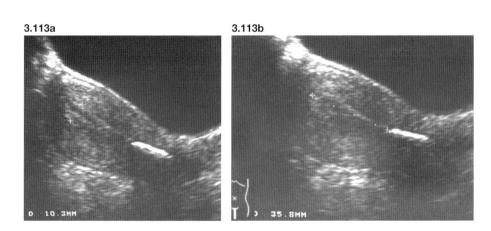

3.113c

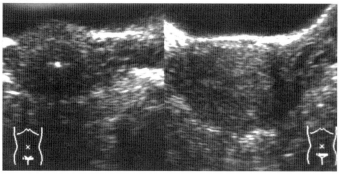

114 This lady in her thirties was referred for a gynaecology scan. She is known to have an irregular cycle of up to 40 days, and has had a gastrectomy. Day 2 scan findings are illustrated in Fig. 3.114. The ovaries were not identified.

a] Describe the ultrasound appearances.

b] What is the likely condition?

c] Is any other non-invasive imaging technique indicated, and why or why not?

d] How may ultrasound be useful in the future management of this lady?

3.114a Uterus 52 × 37 × 29 mm; endometrium 6 mm.

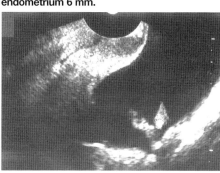

3.114b

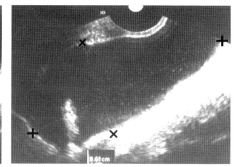

3.114c

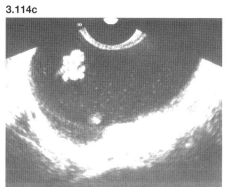

3.114d

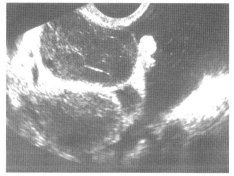

3.114e

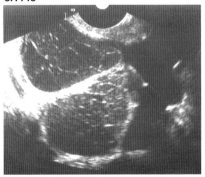

115 This lady in her early thirties was referred with a history of primary infertility. She is known to have up to three menstrual periods a year. Fig. 3.115 illustrates the findings of the day 27 scan. The right ovary (not shown here) had a normal size and echopattern.

a] Describe the ultrasound appearances.

b] What can this condition be?

3.115a

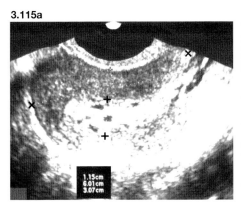

3.115b

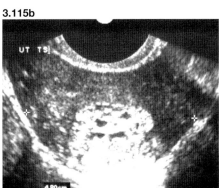

3.115c 44 × 37 × 27 mm.

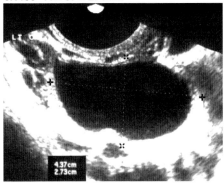

3.116a

3.116b

3.116c

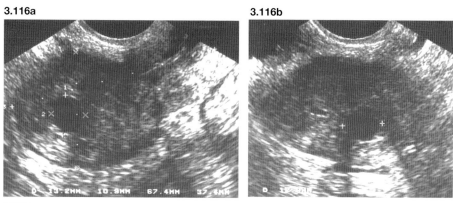

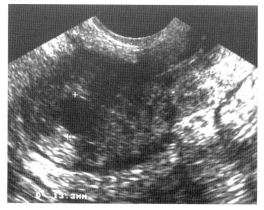

116 This lady was referred because of pelvic pain and dysmenorrhoea. Fig. 3.116 shows the the ultrasound findings of her uterus.
   a] Is the uterine appearance normal or not?
   b] What can this condition be?

117 This long-standing postmenopausal lady was referred for a scan with a history of PV bleeding. The ultrasound findings are illustrated in Fig. 3.117.
   a] Describe the ultrasound appearances.
   b] Where else should the sonographer check and why?
   c] How else can the findings be confirmed?

118 This lady of > 10 years postmenopausal standing was referred for a routine scan. She had never been on HRT. The ultrasound findings are illustrated in Fig. 3.118. The left ovary was not identified; the right ovary appeared normal.
   a] Is there any significant finding in this lady?
   b] Would she require any other investigation, and why or why not?

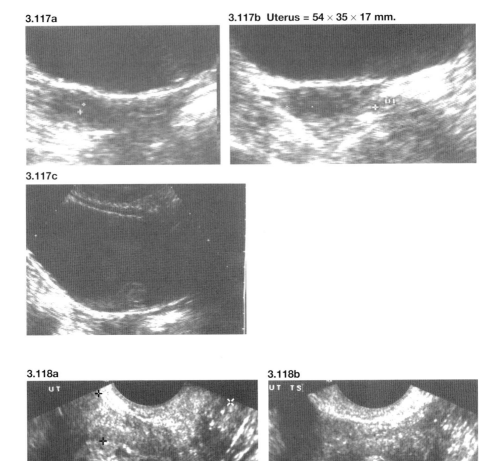

3.117a

3.117b Uterus = 54 × 35 × 17 mm.

3.117c

3.118a

3.118b

119   Fig. 3.119 demonstrates the ultrasound findings of the ovaries of five ladies
      (A–E). Describe the ultrasound appearances in each and the likely condition.
120   Fig. 3.120 illustrates the ultrasound findings of the uterus in each of six ladies
      (A–F). What are the hyperechoic/echogenic structures and where is each located?

3.119a Lady A.

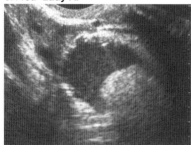

3.119b Lady B. Right ovary = 48 × 41 × 26 mm.

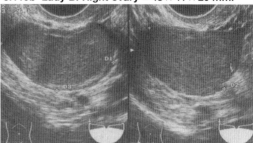

3.119c Lady C. Right ovary = 52 × 33 × 39 mm.

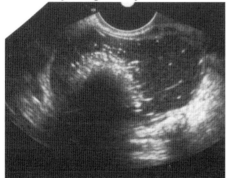

3.119d Lady D. Left ovary 0 = 58 mm, +0 = 49 mm.

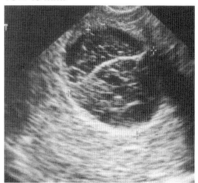

3.119e Lady E.

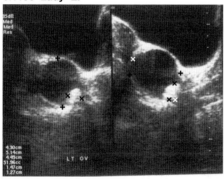

121 This lady of many years postmenopause was referred for a pelvic scan with a history of distended abdomen, breathlessness and loss of weight. The ultrasound findings are shown in Fig. 3.121. The ovaries were not identified.

a] Identify the structures labelled a–e in Fig. 3.121.

b] Describe the ultrasound appearances.

c] Which other non-invasive ultrasound test may be helpful in this lady?

d] Will this lady require any other diagnostic imaging test, and why or why not?

e] How can ultrasound be useful in the future management of this lady?

3.120a Lady A.

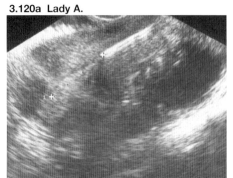

3.120b Lady A.

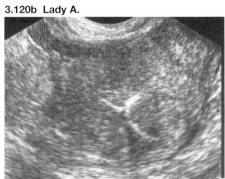

Lady B.

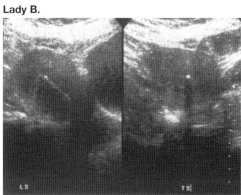

3.120d Lady C.

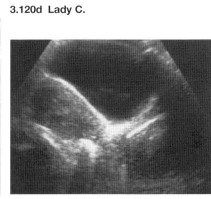

3.120e Lady D.

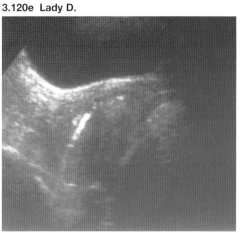

3.120f Lady D.

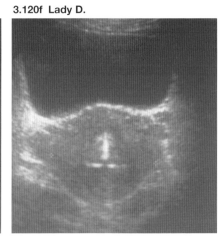

3.120g Lady E.

3.120h Lady E.

3.120i Lady F.

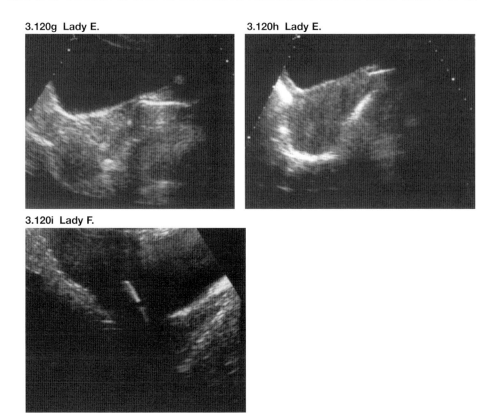

3.121a Right upper quadrant.

3.121b

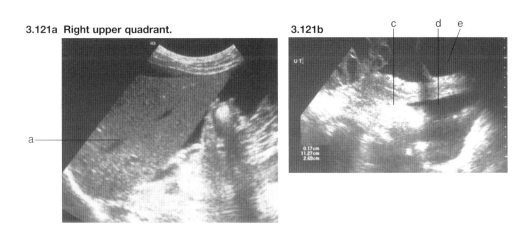

124 Fig. 3.124 illustrates the cervix of a lady.
    a] Describe the ultrasound appearances.
    b] Is there any clinical significance to this finding?
125 This lady was referred because of pelvic pain. The ultrasound findings are illustrated in Fig. 3.125. LMP uncertain but < 6/40 before.
    a] Identify the structures labelled a–d in Fig. 3.125.
    b] Describe the ultrasound appearances.
    c] How may the ultrasound findings be confirmed?
    d] In which way may ultrasound be used in the future management of this patient?
126 This lady was referred with a history of pelvic pain. Fig. 3.126 shows the ultrasound findings.
    a] Describe the ultrasound appearances.
    b] What could this condition be?
    c] In which way may ultrasound be useful in the future management of this patient?

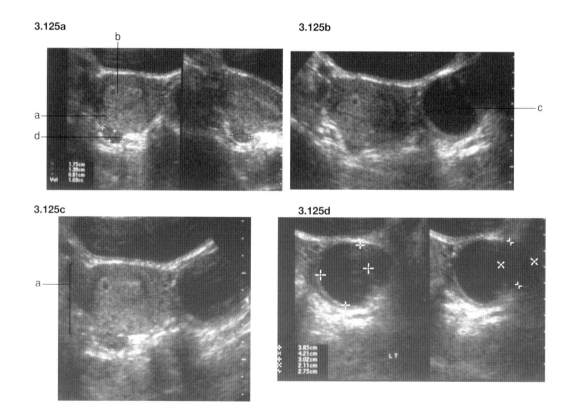

3.125a
3.125b
3.125c
3.125d

3.126a Postmicturition ++ 13 cm.

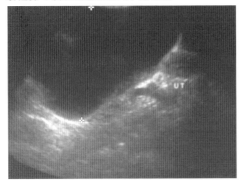

3.126b ++ 4.95 cm.

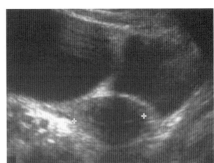

3.126c

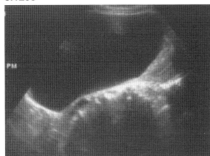

3.126d

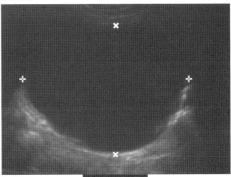

3.126e ++ 18.32 cm.

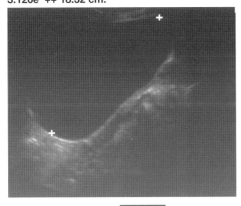

Obstetrics – 1st trimester

LEARNING OBJECTIVES

By the end of working through this chapter the reader should:

- know the two main types of 'bad news' and important points to note when giving patients clinical 'bad news'
- be aware of some clinical indications for 1st trimester scanning
- know how to prepare a patient for 1st trimester or gynaecology scanning
- be aware of the safety of ultrasound on the embryo/fetus
- be aware of how to minimize patient dose during an obstetric scan
- be aware of quality issues as they relate to the 1st trimester scanning programme and in-house quality assurance programmes/clinical audit
- be aware of issues to consider in setting up an Early Pregnancy Unit
- be aware of how to go about patient information leaflet preparation regarding some common medical issues in 1st trimester pregnancy
- be able to date a 1st trimester pregnancy and provide a report of the scan
- understand what an ectopic pregnancy is and its possible ultrasound appearance
- be aware of what a miscarriage is, the various types and ultrasound appearances of a miscarriage and some causes of miscarriage
- know the types and clinical presentations of molar pregnancy and the possible ultrasound findings
- be aware of the use of ultrasound in the clinical staging and follow up of patients with malignant trophoblastic disease
- be aware of the clinical indications, contraindications and possible routes for 1st trimester invasive tests and the possible associated risks
- understand what nuchal thickness screening is, how it is done, what measurements are required, how the risks are calculated and some factors that could affect the calculated risk
- be aware of the causes and the types of multiple pregnancies, ultrasound presentations, reasons for scanning, reporting writing following multiple pregnancy scanning and interpretation of the nuchal translucency screening test in multiple pregnancy
- understand the concept of vanishing or conjoined twins
- in each case presented be able to:
  —identify normal and abnormal ultrasound patterns in the images
  —write an ultrasound report based on the images
  —suggest the possible condition/alternatives
  —suggest which organs/structures should be checked and why
  —understand the implications of the demonstrated conditions
  —be aware of the ultrasound role in the management of the case presented
  —be informed of the presented case outcome where known.

INTRODUCTION

The use of ultrasound scanning as a means of imaging the fetus in utero has caught the public imagination in a manner not typical of medical procedures but as a potentially positive experience for the patient and, for some, a social event in which those close to the patient may be involved. Patients attend the ultrasound department during the 1st trimester of their pregnancy for many reasons. They may have their scans done with or without nuchal thickness (NT) measurement, depending on the existing protocol in the department.

Screening by maternal age and fetal NT at 11–14 weeks of gestation is now proven to identify about 75% of Down's syndrome-affected fetuses with a false positive rate of about 5%. Recent evidence suggests that maternal age can be combined with fetal nuchal thickness and maternal serum biochemistry (free β-hCG) and pregnancy-associated plasma protein (PAPP-A) at 11–14 weeks gestational age to identify about 90% of affected fetuses. However, not all hospitals in United Kingdom offer routine 1st trimester scan to their pregnant women nor perform NT assessment. Many hospitals that perform NT assessment do not have the facilities for conducting the free β-hCG and PAPP-A tests at the same time. Some hospitals do have a dedicated Early Pregnancy Assessment Unit with ultrasound facilities.

◆ Current and future changes within the NHS in the UK may affect practices within obstetric ultrasound departments; for example it is currently unclear whether or not 1st trimester scans with NT screening will become mandatory in the future.

Most people think of breaking bad news in terms of terminal care or death but bad news can also be that which shatters hopes and dreams, and leads perhaps to a very different lifestyle. For parents looking forward to the baby, the threatened loss of pregnancy or fetal death or abnormality can be devastating. Pregnancy being a normal outcome of life, it does not have the buffering that expected disease processes may have in preparing a patient prior to an obstetric ultrasound examination in the same way as when pathology is expected.

Obstetric 'bad news' falls mainly into two types:

- clinical bad news which can be any of the following:
  — unexpected findings during a routine scan (e.g. anembyronic pregnancy, missed abortion, fetal abnormalities)
  — confirmation of expected problems (e.g. due to family history, ectopic pregnancy, poor obstetric history, illness in pregnancy, maternal or clinical suspicion)
- social bad news is that which may bring unexpected trauma to the patient for reasons of personal circumstances (e.g. an unplanned pregnancy or multiple pregnancy).

Some points to consider in breaking clinical bad news:

— there is no easy way of breaking the clinical bad news for the sonographer
— to the patient it is a baby, not an embryo or fetus, so should be referred to as such
— the patient should be given the option of seeing the baby on the screen (this helps the patient to come to terms with the ultrasound findings and later during the grieving process)

— a hard copy of the image of the baby should be offered to the patient/couple and if they refuse at that stage a copy should be made and kept in their hospital notes should they want it later (some find this useful in their grieving process)

— comments such as 'you are young, you can try again' and 'at least you know you can get pregnant' should be avoided. Rather 'we are sorry about this situation' is much preferred.

◆ In ultrasound there are a number of protocols such as the one addressing the written request by the clinician for scanning during the 1st trimester, chaperoning during transvaginal examinations, prescan consent documentation, communicating the scan report (especially in cases of a missed abortion or fetal abnormality), and having husband/children/family present in the scan room during the examination. The sonographer is encouraged to be familiar with departmental protocols such that practice is in line with the agreed hospital protocol.

◆ Obstetric charts used are not the same in all hospitals. While some obstetric ultrasound departments use the recommended British Medical Ultrasound Society (BMUS) charts, other departments may use one of the alternative types of chart available or their own local population-derived charts. As the cases presented here are from various departments, the measurements and subsequent gestational age (GA) depend on the chart used in that particular ultrasound department and this may vary from hospital to hospital.

◆ Unless otherwise stated, in this chapter GA has been worked out accurately in line with the patient's known menstrual cycle.

◆ The format used here in describing the ultrasound appearances may differ from what is used in other hospitals.

QUESTIONS

General questions

1   List the possible clinical indications for 1st trimester scanning.
2   Which ultrasound-recognizable conditions can cause lower abdominal pain in the 1st or 2nd trimester?
3   Which clinical conditions may require urgent ultrasound scan in the 1st trimester?
4   List some ultrasound-recognizable conditions that may be associated with bleeding in early pregnancy.
5   Why do patients need to keep a full bladder for a transabdominal scan (TAS) in the 1st trimester?
6   What is the difference between the patient preparation for TAS and transvaginal scan (TVS) in gynaecology and early pregnancy?
7   Which questions should a sonographer ask the patient before commencing or at beginning of a 1st trimester scan and why?
8   What are some of the causes of early pregnancy failure?
9   What are some of the advantages of the 1st trimester scan?
10   Which points may make moving the 2nd trimester ultrasound anomaly scan to 1st trimester screening difficult at present?

11 How safe is it to perform ultrasound on a 1st trimester embryo/fetus?
12 What precautions can be taken to ensure that the patient dose for an obstetric ultrasound scan is kept to a minimum?
13 In setting up a 1st trimester scanning programme for the ultrasound department, what are some of the quality issues that need to be considered?
14 In setting up an in-house quality assurance programme/clinical audit for the 1st trimester scanning programme, what points should the sonographer bear in mind?
15 An Early Pregnancy Unit (EPU) is being planned for your district general hospital and you have been asked to look into the possibility of having an ultrasound facility within it. What points would you consider?
16 You have been asked to design patient information leaflets for the following conditions which are prevalent in the community where your department is based: anembryonic pregnancy, ectopic pregnancy and hydatidiform mole. In designing these leaflets:
    a] what key issues should be highlighted?
    b] who would you consult and why?
    c] what are the advantages of such information leaflets?

Dating and reporting the 1st trimester scan

17 What is the limitation of the TV approach in obtaining a crown–rump length (CRL)?
18 What factors can lead to obtaining an inaccurate CRL?
19 The LMP is not always reliable for dating a pregnancy. Why?
20 In which women is an error in establishing a LMP highest and why?
21 In which group of women is establishing a LMP difficult?
22 What measurements will you take to date a pregnancy in the 1st trimester?
23 a] What is the earliest ultrasound sign for the confirmation of an intrauterine pregnancy?
    b] The thickening of the endometrium cannot be used as a means of diagnosing pregnancy. Why?
24 a] When and why is the gestational sac volume (GSV) important?
    b] What is the difference between the GSV and the gestational sac diameter (GSD)?
25 How is the GSV calculated?
26 When is the yolk sac seen on ultrasound in pregnancy?
27 When is the body growth most rapid in utero in a normal pregnancy?
28 What is the degree of mathematical error in a CRL measurement?
29 Following a routine 1st trimester scan, what information should the sonographer document?
30 What is the triple test?
31 What are the advantages of a dating scan (DS) prior to the triple test?
32 What is the difference between:
    a] a dating scan
    b] an anomaly scan
    c] a growth scan.

33 Four ladies were referred for a 1st trimester scan on 20/07/97:

Patient	LMP	Cycle
Lady A	21/04/97	24-day regular cycle
Lady B	21/04/97	32–35-day cycle
Lady C	21/04/97	Known irregular cycle, approximately three menstrual periods in a year
Lady D	21/04/97	28–30-day cycle

a] Using the obstetric wheel, calculate the anticipated GA of the fetuses of the four ladies.

b] Give reasons to support the calculated GAs given in Answer 33a.

34 In line with your departmental protocol, briefly outline how you would go about breaking the clinical bad news of a missed abortion of 12 + 5/40 to a couple.

Ectopic pregnancy

35 a] What is an ectopic pregnancy?

b] What are the symptoms which can suggest an ectopic pregnancy?

c] How is the serum hCG level in a patient with a symptomatic ectopic pregnancy different from a patient with a normal intrauterine pregnancy?

d] What is a pseudogestational sac?

e] What causes a pseudogestational sac?

36 a] In the presence of +ve beta hCG > 6500 mIU, which ultrasound findings can suggest an ectopic pregnancy?

b] What are some of the causes of a false-positive diagnosis of ectopic pregnancy with TVS?

37 a] Should the pelvic ultrasound be negative in a patient with a possible ectopic pregnancy, where else should the sonographer check?

b] List the possible ultrasound appearances of an abdominal pregnancy.

38 a] What is the incidence of ectopic pregnancy?

b] Which group of patients is prone to ectopic pregnancy?

c] What is a heterotopic pregnancy?

Miscarriage

39 What is a miscarriage?

40 How can leiomyoma be a cause of recurrent miscarriage?

41 What can cause an incompetent cervix?

42 What is the obstetric significance of an incompetent cervix?

43 Which ultrasound findings are suggestive of an incompetent cervix?

44 Describe the ultrasound types and appearances of an abortion.

Molar pregnancy

45 a] List the possible clinical presentations of a hydatidiform mole in the 1st or 2nd trimester.

  b] What are the different types of molar pregnancy?

  c] What are the ultrasound findings in molar pregnancy?

  d] In some patients with choriocarcinoma, follow-up tests may be required. Which non-laboratory diagnostic tests may be required and why?

  e] Patients who have had a molar pregnancy are advised not to become pregnant while being followed up. Why?

  f] Patients who have had a molar pregnancy are advised not to use contraceptive pills while their hCG values are raised. Why?

  g] What are the chances of a woman who has had a molar pregnancy having another molar pregnancy?

  h] Is a woman who has had chemotherapy for molar pregnancy at an increased risk of abnormal babies in future pregnancies?

46 Which ultrasound findings in the 1st trimester can later progress to hydatidiform mole?

47 What else can mimic a hydatidiform mole in the uterus and how can this structure be differentiated from the mole on ultrasound?

48 List the uses of ultrasound in the clinical staging and follow up of patients with malignant trophoblastic disease.

Others

49 What is the striking ultrasound feature of anencephaly?

50 Why and how can anencephaly be missed?

51 What are Braxton Hicks contractions and how do they differ from the placenta?

52 What are the following, their causes and what effect can they have on the fetus?:
  — amniotic band
  — amniotic sheet
  — unfused amniotic sac
  — subchorionic lucent space.

53 a] What is nuchal cystic hygroma?

  b] In which clinical conditions could cystic hygroma be seen?

54 What clinical condition may be indicated by a large fetal urinary bladder at 12/40?

1st trimester invasive tests

55 What is the difference between CVS and amniocentesis?

56 What is the clinical indication for CVS?

57 What are the contraindications to CVS?

58 What risks can be associated with CVS?

59 List the possible routes for performing CVS and the advantages of each.

60 At what stage of pregnancy can CVS be performed?
61 Apart from the obstetrician, radiographer and midwife, which other person's presence is required at CVS examination and what equipment will the person bring along?
62 What are the advantages and disadvantages of CVS over amniocentesis?
63 What possible technical problems can the obstetrician encounter during CVS?
64 Why is CVS not recommended in multiple pregnancy?
65 List the advantages of direct preparation and culture preparation in chromosomal analysis.
66 What are the disadvantages of direct preparation in CVS?
67 What is the overall risk of pregnancy loss following CVS?
68 In what way may CVS lead to limb deformity and how can this be eliminated?

NT screening

69 What is nuchal thickness (NT) and how is it measured?
70 What is the difference between nuchal thickness and nuchal fold?
71 In the NT screening programme how is the background risk calculated?
72 What is sequential screening?
73 How do the following affect the risk for trisomies?:
  a] maternal age
  b] GA
  c] previous history of a trisomy.
74 How do the following affect the risk for trisomies, for example trisomy 21?:
  a] NT
  b] maternal serum hCG
  c] maternal serum Papanicolaou-A (PAPP-A).
75 How does the GA affect the NT measurement generally in a normal pregnancy?
76 What are the chances of recurrence in a woman with a previous fetus or child with a NTD?

Multiple pregnancy

77 How can the chorionicity of twins be determined on ultrasound in the 1st trimester?
78 What is the difference in the incidence of dizygotic (DZ) and monozygotic (MZ) twins?
79 Genetically how are MZ twins different from DZ twins?
80 What causes conjoined twins?
81 What is the role of ultrasound in the management of conjoined twins?
82 What is the genetic origin of triplets?
83 Why is early diagnosis of twins important?
84 Why is the knowledge of chorionicity and amnionicity important?
85 What is the vanishing twin syndrome?

86 What artefacts may mimic twins on ultrasound during the 1st trimester?

87 Describe the possible ultrasound presentations of twins from one ovum or two ova.

88 What is the amniotic sac membrane?

89 What is the clinical significance of the amniotic sac membrane and why should the sonographer note it in the ultrasound findings?

90 Describe the different membranes seen with twin pregnancy.

91 Which ultrasound features can suggest DZ twins?

92 List some reasons for scanning multiple pregnancy.

93 How does the time of zygote division influence the type of twin?

94 When is the best time to determine chorionicity and why?

95 How is NT screening of twins carried out and interpreted?

Case presentations

96 This patient was referred because of PV bleed for 3 weeks. Previous +ve pregnancy test. GA by known LMP was 10/40. Fig. 4.96 illustrates the ultrasound findings of the uterus. Both ovaries not shown here appeared sonographically normal.

a] Describe the ultrasound appearances.

b] Which possible condition is this?

97 A 26-year-old lady was referred for a scan with a history of hyperemesis and painless PV bleed. GA by LMP at the time of scan was 13/40. Uterine measurement was $106 \times 86 \times 85$ mm. The right ovary (not shown in Fig. 4.97) was $28 \times 24 \times 18$ mm and was normal in echopattern. The left ovary was not identified during that scan.

a] Describe the ultrasound appearances.

b] What is the possible condition demonstrated?

c] Where else should the sonographer check and why?

d] In which way could ultrasound be used in the future management of this lady?

98 Fig. 4.98 shows the ultrasound findings at different GA in two patients following fertility treatments.

a] Describe the ultrasound findings shown in Fig. 4.98.

b] In what ways are the fetuses in Fig. 4.98a and 4.98b different genetically?

4.96

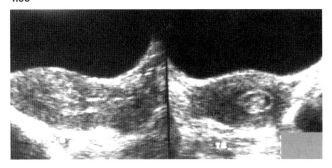

4.97a Longitudinal section.

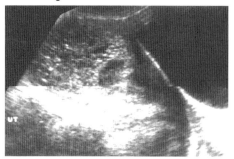

4.97b Transverse section.

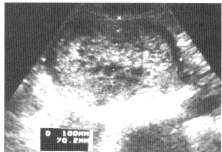

4.97c Fundus magnified.

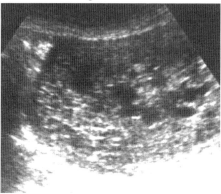

c] Which of the pregnancies is at a higher risk and why?

d] In which ways could ultrasound be used in the future management of these patients?

99 Two ladies, whose uterine ultrasound findings are illustrated in Fig. 4.99, were referred for scan at different GAs. FHB seen in both cases. The ovaries of both ladies (not shown here) appeared normal in size and echopattern.

4.98a Known GA = 6/40. Yolk sacs, fetal poles and FHB were seen.

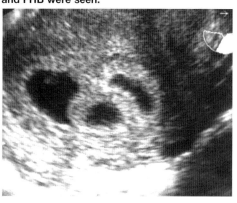

4.98b

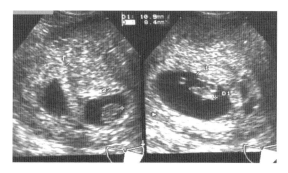

4.99a CRL ≤ 4 mm each; GA by known LMP = 6/40.

4.99b CRL = 9 mm each = date.

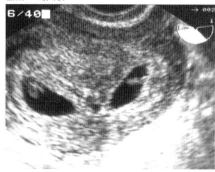

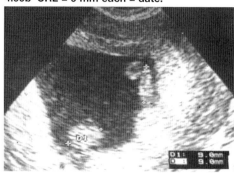

   a] Describe the ultrasound appearances.

   b] Which of these pregnancies is at a higher risk and why?

100   This lady presented with a current medical history of 6/40 light but continuous bleeding. Previous medical history > 10 years of primary infertility.

   CRL = 17 mm = 8 + 3/40 = GA by known embryo transfer (ET) date. FHB and movements were noted. Fig. 4.100 illustrates the ultrasound findings of the uterus.

   a] Describe the ultrasound appearances.

   b] What is the differential diagnosis?

   c] What is the role of ultrasound in the future management of this lady?

   d] 'Can I still miscarry my baby?' the lady asked the sonographer. In line with your departmental protocol, what points should your response highlight?

101   This lady in her twenties was referred because of PV bleed. LMP = 48 days before the scan. +ve pregnancy test result. Fig. 4.101 shows the ultrasound findings of the uterus. CRL = 3 mm. FHB was seen but not demonstrated here.

   a] Write an ultrasound report of the findings in Fig. 4.101.

   b] What are the potential risks in this case?

   c] What is the role of ultrasound in the future management of this lady?

4.100a

4.100b 43 × 24 mm area. Posterior and to the right of GS was B.

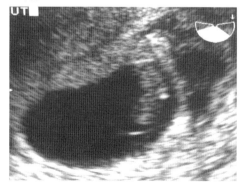

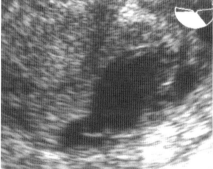

4.101a

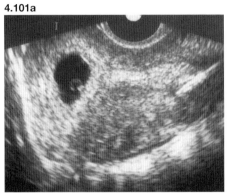

4.101b

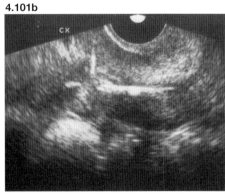

    d] How is an IUCD meant to work to prevent pregnancy?

    e] What is the incidence of pregnancy with an IUCD in situ?

    f] What is the possible reason for the failure of the IUCD to prevent pregnancy in this case?

102   This lady was referred for routine dating scan. GA by known LMP = 8 + 3/40. No history of PV bleeding. Both ovaries and adnexa (not shown here) had normal ultrasound echopatterns. Fig. 4.102 demonstrates the scan findings of the uterus. No FHB was seen.

    a] Describe the ultrasound appearances.

    b] What condition can this be?

    c] What is the role of ultrasound in the future management of this lady?

103   This 37-year-old lady was referred because of bleeding PV for 3/40. GA by LMP = 9 + 1/40. Fig. 4.103 illustrates the scan findings of the uterus. Both ovaries and adnexa (not shown here) had normal ultrasound echopatterns.

4.102

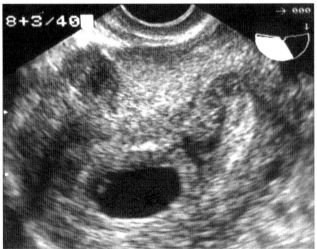

a] Describe the ultrasound appearances.

b] What is the differential diagnosis?

c] What is the role of ultrasound in the future management of this lady?

4.103

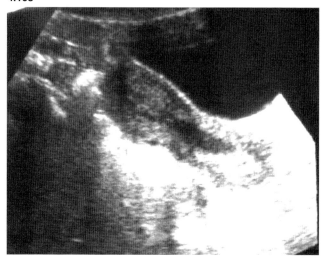

104 This lady was referred because of bleeding PV. LMP unknown. Fig. 4.104 shows the TVS findings of the uterus. Both ovaries and adnexa (not shown here) had normal ultrasound echopatterns. YS (not demonstrated here) was also seen.

a] Describe the ultrasound appearances.

b] What other comment should the sonographer make about the uterus?

c] What is the diagnosis?

d] What is the role of ultrasound in the future management of this lady?

e] How old is this pregnancy approximately, and what could be done to date the pregnancy more accurately in the future?

4.104

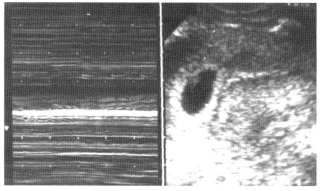

4.105

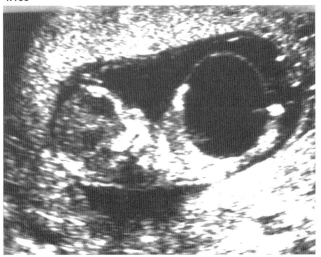

105 This lady was referred for routine 1st trimester scan. Fig. 4.105 illustrates the ultrasound findings. FHB and movements were noted. CRL = dates.
   a] What is the most significant ultrasound finding?
   b] Where could this finding originate?
   c] In what way could this finding affect the pregnancy?

106 This lady was referred because of slight bleeding PV. LMP = 8/40 ago. Fig. 4.106 illustrates the scan findings of the uterus, CRL was 20 mm = 8/40 and FHB was seen. Both ovaries and adnexa (not shown here) had normal ultrasound echopatterns.
   a] What is the difference between Fig. 4.106a and 4.106b? Write an ultrasound report of the findings in Fig. 4.106.
   b] What is the differential diagnosis?
   c] What is the effect of a full bladder on this type of uterus for an early TA pregnancy scan?

4.106a   **4.106b**

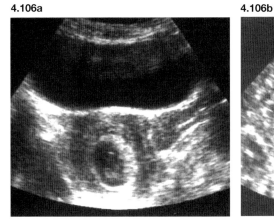
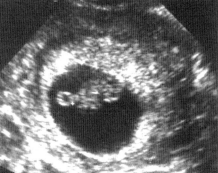

107 This lady in her thirties was referred for a scan. She had red blood bleeding for a
week before the scan. Positive pregnancy test. GA by known LMP ~ 6+/40.
Previous left salpingectomy for left ectopic pregnancy.
a] Describe the ultrasound appearances in Fig. 4.107.
b] What is the differential diagnosis?
c] How can this finding affect this lady's future ability to conceive?

4.107a ++ = 8.8 mm.

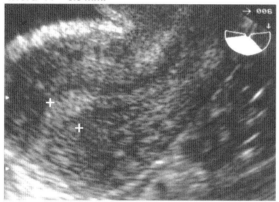

4.107b 15 mm.

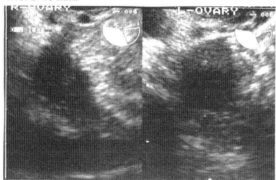

4.107c

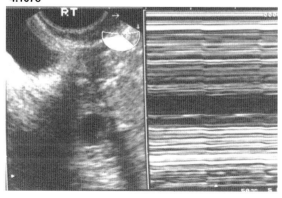

4.107d Right adnexus.

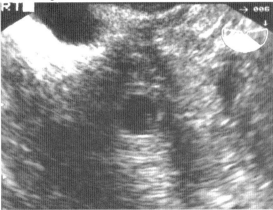

108 This 24-year-old lady is on the combined oral contraceptive pill. LMP = 6+/40 before. +ve pregnancy home kit test but had abnormal bleeding for a few days before this scan. Fig. 4.108 illustrates the ultrasound findings.

4.108a Right side.

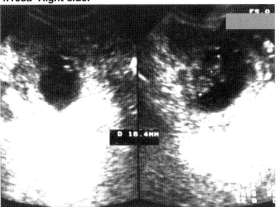

4.108b

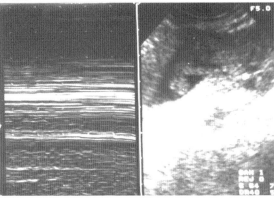

4.108c

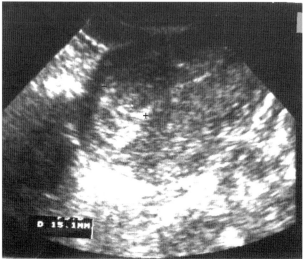

4.108d

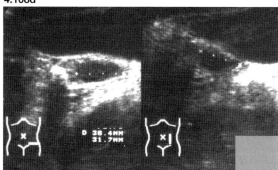

4.109

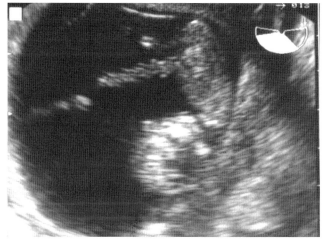

a] Describe the above ultrasound appearances.
b] What are the differential diagnoses?
c] How does the progesterone-only pill work?
d] Which factors can contribute to a woman getting pregnant while on the pill?

109 Fig. 4.109 shows a fetus at 11 + 3/40. As the NT cannot be measured in this position, what can the sonographer do in order to obtain the NT measurement?

110 A 1st trimester scan at 12/40 revealed the findings in Fig. 4.110. CRL = GA by LMP. FHB and movements were seen.
a] Write an ultrasound report.
b] What are the differential diagnoses?
c] How may ultrasound be used in the future management of this patient?

111 Fig. 4.111 illustrates the ultrasound findings of the uterus during a routine 1st trimester scan. GA by known LMP = 12/40. CRL = 55 mm = 12 + 1/40. FHB and movements were seen.
a] Write an ultrasound report.
b] Which invasive diagnostic test could be offered to this lady at this GA and what information could be obtained from the test?

4.110a   **4.110b**

4.110c   **4.110d**

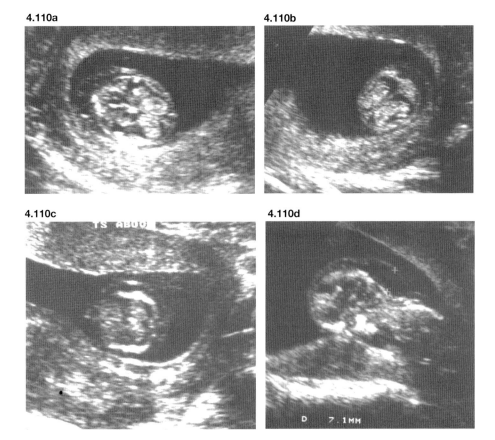

4.110e

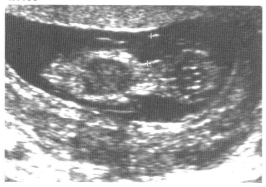

4.111a

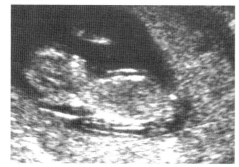

4.111b ++ = 5.4 mm.

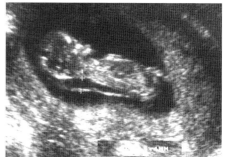

4.112 ++ = 4.7 mm.

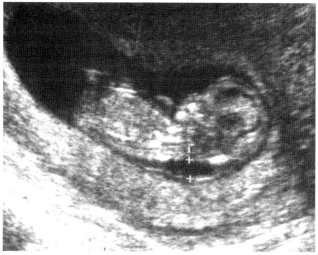

112 Fig. 4.112 illustrates the ultrasound findings of the uterus in a woman in her twenties during a routine 1st trimester scan. FHB and movements were noted. CRL = 51 mm = 11 + 6/40 = dates. Normal adnexa were seen.
a] Describe the ultrasound appearances.
b] CVS demonstrated a normal karyotype. Which other ultrasound diagnostic test can be offered to this lady and why?

4.113a

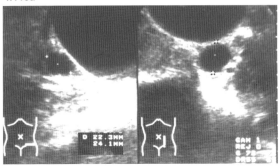

4.113b

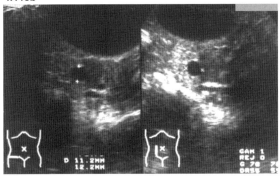

4.113c

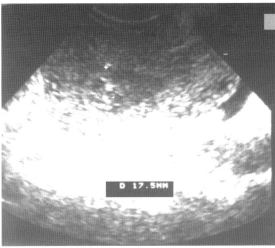

113   This lady was referred for a scan because of continuous PV bleed following
        evacuation of retained products of conception (ERPC). There is a recent medical
        history of a hydatidiform mole. Fig. 4.113 shows the ultrasound findings.
        a] Describe the ultrasound appearances.
        b] Where else should the sonographer check and why?

114   Fig. 4.114 illustrates the findings during a routine 1st trimester scan.
        CRL = 32 mm = 10 + 1/40. YS, FHB and movements (not shown here) were seen.
        a] Identify the structures labelled i–v in Fig. 4.114.
        b] Is structure ii a normal finding at this stage and how does the GA affect this
           finding?

115   Fig. 4.115 shows the ultrasound findings of the uterus during a routine 1st
        trimester scan. GA by known LMP = 12 + 0/40.
        a] Write an ultrasound report.
        b] What is the clinical condition?

4.114a

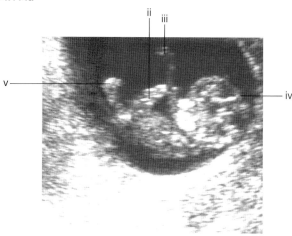

4.114b

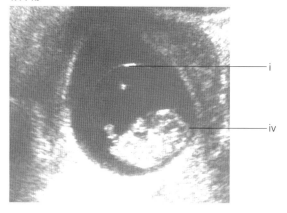

4.115a ++ = 18 mm = 8 + 1/40.

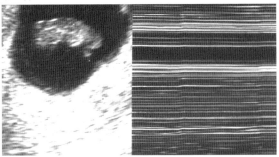

4.115b

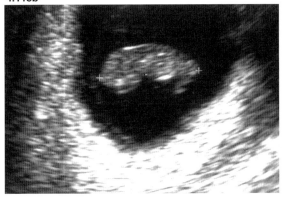

116 This lady was referred for a 1st trimester scan. Fig. 4.116 shows the ultrasound findings of the uterus.

    a] Describe the ultrasound appearances.

    b] Which type of twins is seen in Fig. 4.116?

    c] What condition is this?

    d] What is the possible effect of sac 2 on sac 1?

117 Fig. 4.117 illustrates the ultrasound finding during a routine 1st trimester scan. FHB and movements were seen.

    a] Describe the ultrasound appearances.

    b] What entity is seen indenting the GS and how can one be sure of the diagnosis?

118 This lady was referred because of previous PV bleeding. GA by LMP = 11 + 4/40. Fig. 4.118 demonstrates the findings of the uterus. CRL = 49 mm = 11 + 3/40; CRL = 50 mm = 11 + 4/40. FHB and movements were seen in both sacs.

    a] Describe the ultrasound appearances.

    b] What are the differential diagnoses?

    c] What is the role of ultrasound in the future management of this lady?

4.116a CRL = 15 mm.

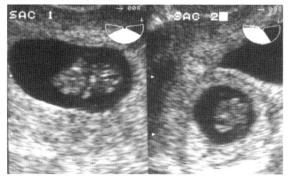

4.116b CRL = 20 mm.

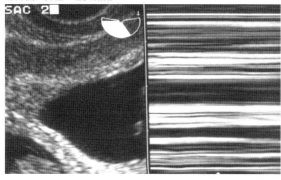

4.116c

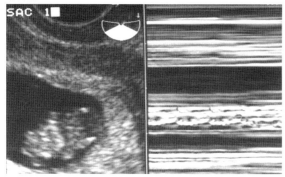

119 This lady in her early twenties was referred for a scan with a history of spotting. She informed the sonographer at the beginning of the scan 'this is a much-wanted pregnancy, I just hope everything is fine'. Previous history of a TOP some years before. GA by known LMP = 8 + 1/40. YS (not demonstrated here) was seen. Fig. 4.119 illustrates the ultrasound finding of her uterus.

a] Describe the ultrasound findings of the uterus.

b] When she was informed of the scan findings she was upset about the result and kept saying 'I am being punished'. Why is this?

4.117

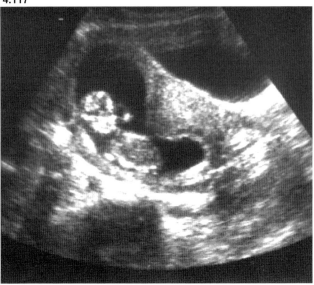

4.118a ++ = 63 × 45 × 11 mm.

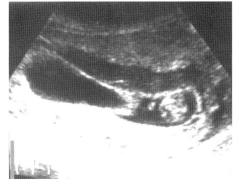

4.118b

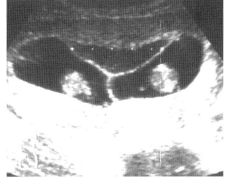

4.119

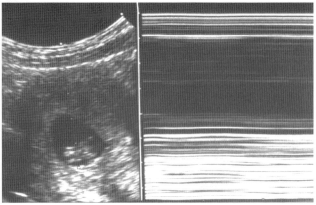

120 This lady in her early twenties was referred for a routine 1st trimester scan. Fig. 4.120 illustrates the ultrasound findings of the uterus and ovaries. FHB and movements were seen. CRL = 33 mm = 10 + 2/40; CRL = 32 mm = 10 + 1/40.
   a] Write an ultrasound report on the findings in Fig. 4.120.
   b] In order to interpret the ultrasound appearance of the ovaries, what question should the sonographer ask the patient and why?
   c] What is the role of ultrasound in the future management of this lady?

121 This lady was referred for a routine 1st trimester scan. Fig. 4.121 illustrates the ultrasound findings of the uterus. FHB and movements were seen. CRL = 53 mm = 12/40 = date.
   a] Identify the structures labelled a–e in Fig. 4.121, name the views and what each view demonstrates.
   b] What is structure b and is it a normal finding at this GA?
   c] List the medical conditions that may be associated with this finding.
   d] What causes this defect?

122 The views in Fig. 4.122 were taken during a 1st trimester scan in two different patients.
   a] Identify the views in Fig. 4.122 and indicate what each view demonstrates.
   b] Which clinical conditions can be ruled out in Fig. 4.122c?

4.120a

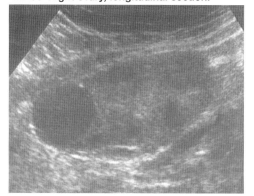

4.120b Left ovary, longitudinal section.

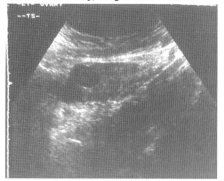

4.120c Right ovary, longitudinal section.

4.120d Right ovary, transverse section.

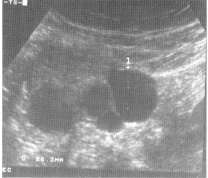

4.121a

4.121b

4.121c

4.121d

4.121e

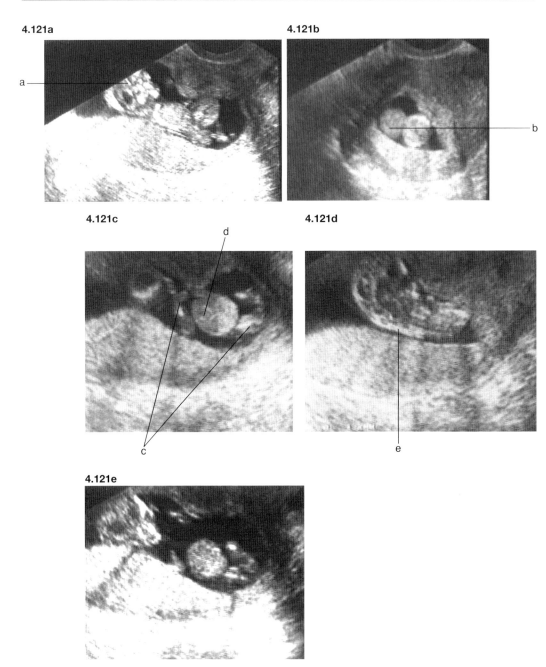

123 This 26-year-old lady was referred because of PV bleed. LMP unsure, +ve
pregnancy test. Fig. 4.123 demonstrates the TVS findings.
CRL = 14 mm = 7 + 5/40. GSD = 33 mm = 8 + 5/40.
a] Describe the ultrasound findings in Fig. 4.123.
b] What are the differential diagnoses?

4.122a

4.122b

4.122c

4.122d

4.122e

4.122f

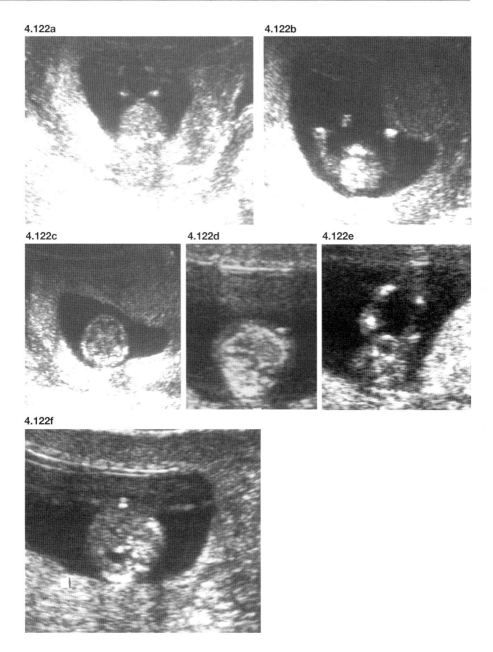

124 This 23-year-old lady was referred because of slight PV bleed with no associated pain. LMP unsure. YS and FHB (not demonstrated in Fig. 4.124) were seen. CRL = 7 mm = 6 + 4/40.

a] Identify the hypoechoic area anterior to the gestational sac.

b] What may cause this ultrasound appearance?

c] What is the role of ultrasound in the management of this lady?

4.123a

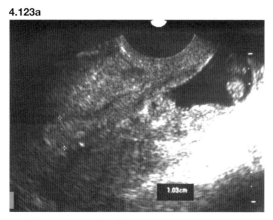

4.123b 1.41 cm = 7w 6d

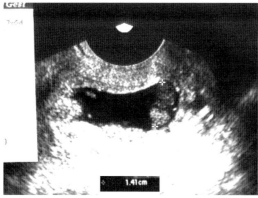

4.123c

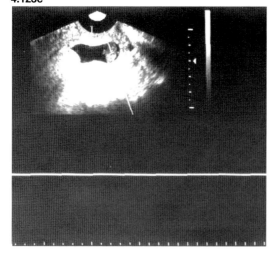

125   This 27-year-old lady was referred for a dating scan. LMP unknown. No history
of PV bleed or pelvic pain. Past history of secondary infertility for over 5 years.
a] Describe the ultrasound findings in Fig. 4.125.

4.124

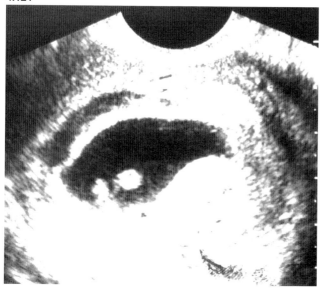

4.125a CRL = 15.4 mm = 7 + 6/40.

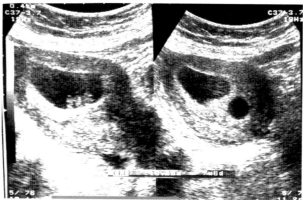

4.125b

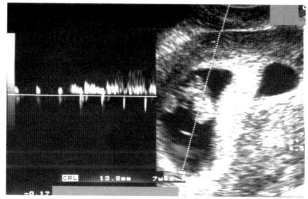

135 This lady presented with PV bleed and pain. LMP 6/40, +ve pregnancy test. Both ovaries (not shown in Fig. 4.135) appeared sonographically normal and a 12 × 10 mm CLC was noted in the left ovary.
   a] Describe the ultrasound findings.
   b] Calculate the GSV in this pregnancy.
   c] What is the likely condition and why?
   d] Which other observation during the scan may help in assessing findings?

136 This lady was referred because of PV discharge. LMP 40 days before. Fig. 4.136a illustrates the ultrasound findings in this patient.
   a] Describe the ultrasound findings.
   b] In which way is the ultrasound appearance in Fig. 4.136a different from that of another patient in Fig. 4.136b?

137 Routine 1st trimester scan. This lady is known to have an irregular cycle, up to two periods in a year. LMP = 82 days before, +ve pregnancy test. PV bleed denied. Fig. 4.137 illustrates the ultrasound findings of the uterus.
   a] Describe the ultrasound findings.
   b] How should these findings be interpreted?

138 Fig. 4.138 illustrates a routine 1st trimester scan.
   a] Describe the significant finding in the placenta.
   b] What could this finding be?
   c] How may ultrasound be used in the future management of this patient?

4.135a

4.135b 36 × 18 × 17 mm.

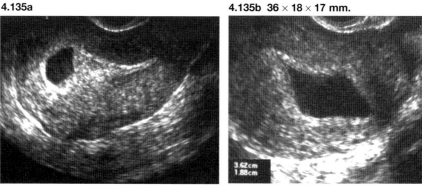

4.135c

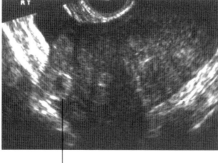

7 mm × 7 mm × 9 mm

4.136a

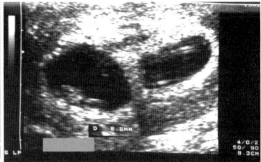

4.136b Fetal heart beats × 2 seen.

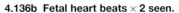

4.137a ++ = 39 × 27 × 24 mm.

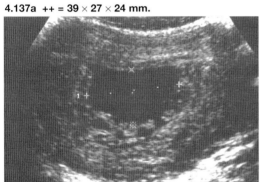

4.137b

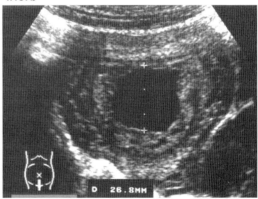

4.138a

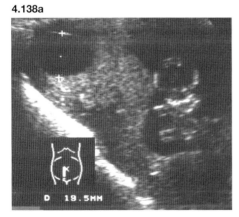

4.138b

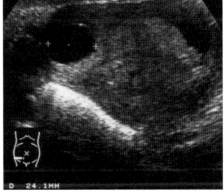

139 This lady was referred for a scan at 13/40. Fig. 4.139 shows the ultrasound findings.
   a] Write an ultrasound report.
   b] What is the possible differential diagnosis?

140. Fig. 4.140 illustrates the findings of a scan at 12/40. CRL was 1/40 < GA by LMP.
   a] Write an ultrasound report.
   b] What are the possible differential diagnoses?

4.139a

4.139d

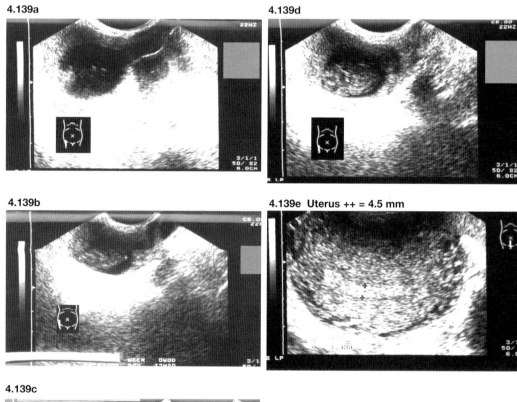

4.139b

4.139e Uterus ++ = 4.5 mm

4.139c

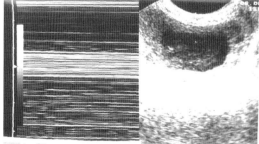

141. This lady was scanned at 12/40. Fig. 4.141 illustrates the ultrasound findings. CRL = dates. FHB and movements were seen. No previous bleed.
    a] Write an ultrasound report.
    b] What is the possible differential diagnosis?
    c] How may ultrasound be used in the future management of this patient?
142. Fig. 4.142 shows an image taken during a 1st trimester screening test.
    a] How was this lady scanned?
    b] What are the measurements?
    c] What are your observations on the screening test and what should be done?

4.140a

4.140b

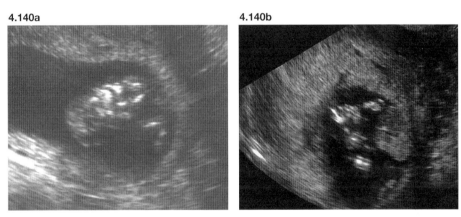

4.140c

4.140d

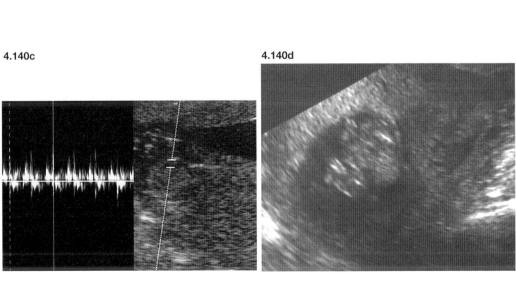

4.141a

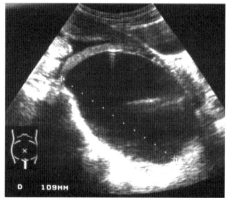

4.141b

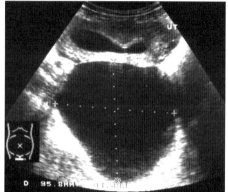

4.141c

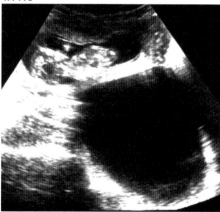

4.142

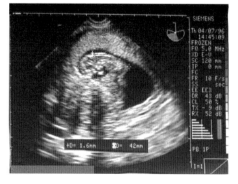

Obstetrics – 2nd and 3rd trimester, part one

LEARNING OBJECTIVES

By the end of working through this chapter the reader should:

- be aware of what could make communicating obstetric clinical 'bad news' stressful for the sonographer and how to minimize such stress
- be aware of the possible clinical indications for 2nd and 3rd trimester scanning
- be able to date a 2nd or 3rd trimester pregnancy and provide a report of the scan
- be aware of clinical indications, contraindications and possible routes for 2nd and 3rd trimester invasive tests and the possible associated risks
- be able to assess and measure the fetal anatomy in the 2nd and 3rd trimester
- know how to assess the fetal urinary tract and gender
- be aware of some common fetal urinary tract problems
- be aware of some common fetal problems
- know how to assess the placenta and amniotic fluid
- be aware of ultrasound 'soft markers' and their implications
- be aware of some chromosomal abnormalities and related problems
- know a normal growth pattern
- be able to assess fetal presentation in the 2nd and 3rd trimester
- be able to identify an abnormal growth pattern, its types and implications
- be aware of some maternal problems in pregnancy
- be aware of possible problems associated with multiple pregnancy and the need for serial ultrasound scans
- be aware of the ultrasound appearances of intrauterine death in the 2nd or 3rd trimester
- be able to identify some structures in a normal fetal heart
- be aware of suspicious abnormal heart size or chest size
- be aware of fetal tachycardia or bradycardia
- be aware of the ultrasound features of the normal fetal left ventricular/fetal right ventricular outflow tracts
- be aware of what pericardial effusion is and its possible ultrasound appearances
- in each case presented be able to:
  - —date the pregnancy/pregnancies
  - —write an ultrasound report and plot the graphs from the information obtained
  - —suggest the possible condition/alternatives
  - —understand the implications of the ultrasound findings
  - —be aware of the ultrasound role in the management of the case presented
  - —be informed of the presented case outcome where known.

INTRODUCTION

The diagnosis of fetal anomalies by ultrasound and consequently how this affects obstetric management were initially authenticated in the early 1970s. Since then, ultrasound diagnosis of structural fetal abnormalities and prenatal management have become an essential and advancing part of prenatal diagnosis and therapy.

Many fetal abnormalities can now be diagnosed with near certainty. For others, such as those associated with intrauterine infection or exposure to potentially teratogenic drugs, only a probability of abnormality can be provided.

The purpose of antenatal screening procedures inclusive of ultrasound examinations is not intended to minimize the occurrence of handicap or to save the resources necessary for the support of handicapped individuals. It is rather aimed at providing the couple with accurate information about the fetus so that they have a choice to give birth to a seriously handicapped child or to have the pregnancy terminated.

Results of all antenatal screening procedures including ultrasound examination (whether negative or positive), when communicated to the couple sensitively, clearly and without delay, eliminates patient distress. Organized and early follow-up appointments with the consultant or referral centre is helpful.

◆ Obstetric charts used are not the same in all hospitals. While some obstetric ultrasound departments use the recommended British Medical Ultrasound Society (BMUS) charts, other departments may use one of the alternative types of chart available or their own local population-derived charts. As the cases presented here are from various departments, the measurements and subsequent gestational age (GA) depend on the chart used in that particular ultrasound department and this may vary from hospital to hospital.

◆ Unless otherwise stated, in this chapter GA has been worked out accurately in line with the patient's known menstrual cycle.

◆ The format used here in describing the ultrasound appearances may differ from what is used in other hospitals.

◆ The sonographer is encouraged to be familiar with departmental protocols such that practice is in line with the agreed hospital protocol.

QUESTIONS
General questions

1 a] List some of the circumstances which could make communicating obstetric clinical 'bad news' stressful for the sonographer.
  b] How could the sonographer's stress at breaking clinical 'bad news' be minimized?
2 List the possible clinical indications for 2nd trimester scanning.
3 List the possible clinical indications for 3rd trimester scanning.
4 a] Which groups of women are more susceptible to preterm labour and delivery?
  b] List some of the clinical indications for ultrasound assessment of the cervix.

    c] Which methods can be used in assessing the cervix and what are the advantages, disadvantages and limitations of each?

    d] Describe the transvaginal scan (TVS) method of assessing the cervix.

    e] In assessing the cervix, what are the things to note?

    f] What are some of the risks associated with cervical cerlage?

5 What problems may fibroids cause in pregnancy?

6 For which clinical conditions can TVS be required in the 3rd trimester?

7 Which clinical conditions may require urgent ultrasound in the 2nd or 3rd trimester?

8 What are the possible causes of 2nd or 3rd trimester bleeding?

9 In which clinical conditions can there be lower abdominal pain in the 3rd trimester?

10 List at least seven possible clinical indications for ultrasound after 24 weeks GA.

11 What is the supine hypotension syndrome and how can this be avoided?

12 What factors could make a pregnancy a 'high-risk' pregnancy?

13 For each of the following drugs/teratogens identify the critical period when a fetus could be affected and the possible ultrasound-identifiable malformation: alcohol, cytomegalovirus, lithium, phenytoin hydantoin, rubella, sodium valproate, thalidomide, toxoplasmosis, varicella (chickenpox), warfarin.

14 Which diagnostic techniques may be used in utero?

Dating and reporting the 2nd/3rd trimester scan

15 Following a non-anomaly 2nd or 3rd trimester scan, what information should the sonographer document?

16 Following a non-anomaly 2nd trimester scan of a multiple pregnancy, what information should the sonographer document?

17 a] Which fetal measurements should be taken routinely after 14 weeks GA?

    b] What is the difference between the charts that are used for dating and the ones used for assessing fetal growth?

    c] What is the difference between a plotted chart and a derived chart, and what is their significance?

18 a] What is an ultrasound 'soft marker'?

    b] What is the clinical significance of an ultrasound soft marker?

    c] List some soft markers.

    d] What are some of the advantages of having an agreed fetal medicine unit (FMU) where patients can be referred for a second opinion?

    e] When a fetal abnormality is discovered in your hospital, which organization will need to be informed?

    f] For how long should obstetric reports be kept?

    g] What are the basic requirements for those performing obstetric ultrasound scans in the UK?

    h] What are some of the medicolegal issues in the UK which the sonographer should be aware of in clinical practice?

19 What is a 'golf ball' and what is its clinical significance?

Invasive procedures

20 a] What is the difference between CVS and amniocentesis?
   b] List some of the clinical indications for amniocentesis.
   c] What risks can be associated with amniocentesis?
   d] What are the advantages and disadvantages of a detailed scan compared to amniocentesis?
   e] What is the overall risk of performing amniocentesis?

21 a] What is cordocentesis and when is it commonly performed?
   b] List the possible clinical indications for cordocentesis.
   c] Which fetal structure should the sonographer identify prior to cordocentesis?
   d] What possible technical problems can the obstetrician encounter during cordocentesis?
   e] What is the overall risk of performing cordocentesis?

22 a] What is AFP?
   b] How is AFP excreted?
   c] When is AFP in the fetal blood at its peak?
   d] What is the significance of the maternal AFP result?
   e] List the ultrasound-recognizable factors that could lead to an inaccurate maternal AFP result.
   f] Which non-ultrasound-identifiable reasons could lead to an incorrect MSAFP result?
   g] Which ultrasound-identifiable conditions should be suspected in a patient with a raised MSAFP?
   h] Why is the AFP assay measurement higher in fetuses with open NTDs, gastroschisis and omphalocele?

23 a] List the duties of the sonographer prior to an amniocentesis.
   b] List the after-care duties of the sonographer and outline the advice the patient may be given following amniocentesis.

24 Why is it important to know the maternal Rhesus factor before an amniocentesis?

25 Why is amniocentesis performed between 16 and 18 weeks GA?

26 Where an amniocentesis is performed to investigate a Rhesus problem, which special equipment is required and why?

27 a] List the instruments needed for CVS.
   b] List the instruments needed for amniocentesis.
   c] List the instruments needed for cordocentesis.

Fetal anatomy assessment and measurements

28 List the ultrasound normal position and appearance of the following fetal structures:
   — stomach
   — spleen
   — liver
   — gall bladder

 — kidneys
 — urinary bladder
 — cord insertion
 — bowels.

29 On a routine 18–20 weeks anomaly scan list the essential fetal anatomy that should be checked.

30 a] In which planes should the fetal facial face be checked and what can be seen in each plane?
   b] Why should the fetal facial structures be checked?
   c] Which possible ultrasound-recognizable mass(es) can arise from the fetal face?

31 a] List the planes for examining the fetal spine and describe its normal appearance.
   b] When examining the fetal spine, which spinal abnormalities are best demonstrated in each plane?

32 What is the typical shape of the cervical spine in the longitudinal section (LS)?

33 Describe how the ossification centres appear in the fetal spine in each plane.

34 a] What does spina bifida refer to?
   b] Which ultrasound appearances are suggestive of spina bifida?
   c] Why are fetuses with open spina bifida able to move their limbs and urinate in utero?
   d] What is the difference between spina bifida and anencephaly?
   e] What is the incidence of NTD?

35 Which ultrasound fetal spine appearances are indicative of myelomeningocele?

36 How is encephalocele different from cystic hygroma on ultrasound?

37 Which thoracic structures should be checked during the anomaly scan?

38 a] Describe the ultrasound appearances of the normal fetal lungs.
   b] Which clinical conditions can make the fetal lungs appear more echogenic on ultrasound?

39 a] List the brain structures that may be checked in the 18–20 weeks anomaly scan.
   b] Which fetal anomalies can be excluded by visualizing a normal cavum septum pellucidum?
   c] Which fetal anomalies can be excluded by visualizing and having a normal ventricular measurement?
   d] Which fetal anomalies can be excluded by a normal cerebellum and cisterna magna?
   e] What is the normal diameter of the cisterna magna?
   f] What is mild ventriculomegaly?
   g] In which clinical condition is the fetal cisterna magna not easily identified?
   h] When is the 4th ventricle seen?
   i] Which ultrasound appearance can be suggestive of ventriculomegaly?

40 a] On which section should the nuchal fold (NF) be measured at the anomaly scan and how?
   b] What is the normal range of this measurement and what is the clinical significance if it is greater than the range?

41 a] On which section is the BPD measured and how?
    b] List the possible factors that can lead to an inaccurate BPD.
    c] What problems can affect BPD measurement, especially in late pregnancy?
    d] How accurate is the BPD measurement in dating GA in the 2nd trimester?
    e] How accurate is the BPD measurement in dating GA in the 3rd trimester?
    f] What is the difference between dolichocephaly and brachycephaly?
    g] Why is the BPD not used for growth assessment in the 3rd trimester?

42 a] On which section is the HC measured and how may this be done?
    b] In which patients are the BPD and HC measurements important to the obstetrician in the 2nd or 3rd trimester?
    c] In which section should the fetal head be assessed for strawberry shape?
    d] In which clinical conditions can a strawberry-shaped head be seen?

43 What is the shape of a normal fetal cerebellum?

44 a] What is a choroid plexus cyst (CPC)?
    b] What is an isolated choroid plexus cyst (ICPC)?
    c] Discuss the clinical significance of choroid plexus cyst and what action may be taken.
    d] What is the difference on ultrasound between a choroid plexus cyst and a porencephalic cyst?
    e] What is the dangling choroid plexus and what is its clinical significance?

45 a] What does the AVHR ratio represent?
    b] On which section is the AVHR measured?
    c] How is the AVHR ratio measured?
    d] What is the normal average of the AVHR at 18 weeks GA?

46 a] Which ultrasound findings can raise the possibility of fetal hydrocephaly?
    b] How is the diagnosis of hydrocephaly made on ultrasound?
    c] List the types of hydrocephaly and their possible causes.
    d] What is isolated hydrocephaly?
    e] Ultrasonically, when can sex-linked hydrocephaly be ruled out in a woman with a previous affected fetus?

47 a] What is microcephaly?
    b] Which ultrasound findings can indicate a possible fetal microcephaly?
    c] What causes microcephaly?
    d] How may microcephaly be missed on ultrasound?

48 a] List the possible causes of ventriculomegaly.
    b] List the ultrasound signs of ventriculomegaly.
    c] How is hydrocephalus different from ventriculomegaly?

49 a] What is the cephalic index (ci)?
    b] When is the ci used and what is its significance?

50 What are the points in favour of ultrasound at 16–20 weeks GA?

51 a] What is the significance of the stomach bubble?
    b] In which clinical conditions is the double bubble appearance seen?
    c] In which clinical conditions is the triple bubble appearance seen?

52 Which ultrasound findings would make you suspect fetal:
    a] oesophageal atresia?
    b] jejunoileal atresia or anal atresia?
53 What is the difference between duodenal atresia and choledochal cyst?
54 How does jejunal atresia present on ultrasound?
55 What is an omphalocele and how does this present on ultrasound?
56 What is the difference between an omphalocele and gastroschisis?
57 What is the difference between omphalocele and body stalk abnormality?
58 Which fetal conditions can be ruled out by the transverse section (TS) showing the cord insertion?
59 a] Umbilical hernia may be easily missed on a single ultrasound scan. Why?
    b] How does umbilical hernia present on ultrasound?
60 Which ultrasound features are suggestive of diaphragmatic hernia?
61 Which ultrasound appearances of the fetal bowel may be suggestive of bowel obstruction?
62 List the possible ultrasound features that may suggest prune belly anomaly.
63 Which fetal ultrasound appearances may be associated with cystic fibrosis?
64 a] On which section is the abdominal circumference (AC) measured and how?
    b] What problems can affect AC measurement, especially in late pregnancy?
    c] List the possible reasons for obtaining an inaccurate AC.
    d] What is the effect of an anteriorly placed spine when obtaining the AC section?
    e] Why is it important that the AC be measured at the level of the stomach and portal hook?
    f] Which fetal organ can be confused with the portal vein on the section on which the AC is measured?
65 What is the permissible margin of error in ultrasound measurement?

Urinary tract and fetal gender

66 What is the normal fetal kidney circumference to abdominal circumference ratio (KC:AC)?
67 a] Which urinary tract conditions may be suspected/confirmed by ultrasound prenatally?
    b] When a renal anomaly is seen on routine fetal scan what other information should the sonographer document?
    c] What are some of the advantages of antenatal monitoring of renal anomalies by ultrasound?
68 What is the ultrasound difference between an infantile polycystic kidney and a multicystic kidney?
69 a] Which ultrasound features are indicative of bilateral renal agenesis?
    b] Why could unilateral renal agenesis be missed on ultrasound?
    c] How can renal agenesis be differentiated from fetal adrenal glands on ultrasound?

70 How can severe obstructive uropathy (e.g. urethral stenosis or atresia) be differentiated from bilateral renal agenesis on ultrasound?

71 a] What is multicystic kidney disease?
   b] Which ultrasound features can suggest multicystic kidney disease?

72 a] What is infantile polycystic kidney disease?
   b] Which ultrasound features may suggest infantile polycystic kidney disease?

73 a] Which ultrasound appearance may be indicative of pelvic ureteric junction obstruction (PUJO)?
   b] How can PUJO be differentiated from multicystic kidney disease (MKD) on ultrasound?

74 For which clinical conditions is prenatal confirmation of the fetal gender necessary?

75 What are some of the points for and against telling the parents the fetal sex during the routine anomaly scan?

76 Which clinical conditions are suggested by bilateral hydrocele?

Placenta and amniotic fluid

77 a] What are the characteristic ultrasound appearances of fetal hydrops?
   b] List some classifications of fetal hydrops.
   c] In which clinical conditions can fetal skin oedema be seen on ultrasound?

78 a] What is the ultrasound appearance of the placenta at 16–20 weeks GA?
   b] What is placenta praevia?
   c] Why is the term placenta praevia not used before 28 weeks GA?
   d] How may placenta praevia be evaluated?
   e] What is the Braxton Hicks contraction and how does it differ from the placenta?
   f] How does a Braxton Hicks contraction differ from a fibroid?

79 What is a chorioangioma?

80 Where a placental tumour is seen on ultrasound, what else should the sonographer note about the fetus and why?

81 What are the following and what is their clinical significance?:
   — succenturiate lobe
   — placental lake
   — placental cyst
   — highly echogenic areas within the placenta.

82 a] What is placental abruption?
   b] What is the role of ultrasound in the management of placental abruption?
   c] What is placenta percreta?

83 In patients with previous caesarean section, what other information should the sonographer note about the placenta?

84 What is the clinical significance of placenta circumvallata?

85 Why is placenta monitoring essential in a Rhesus -ve pregnant mother?

86 What is the vernix?

87 What is the amniotic band syndrome (ABS)?

88 a] List and describe the non-invasive methods of assessing the amniotic fluid volume.

b] What are the advantages of ultrasound assessment of the amniotic fluid volume?

c] What are the limitations of the ultrasound assessment of the amniotic fluid volume?

89 a] What is the amniotic fluid index (AFI)?

b] How is the AFI measured?

c] What is the clinical significance of the AFI?

d] What is the average liquor volume?

e] What is the absence of any measurable amniotic fluid called?

90 a] What is the difference between anhydramnios, oligohydramnios and polyhydramnios?

b] In which clinical conditions can polyhydramnios be seen on ultrasound?

c] Which ultrasound-recognizable conditions can be responsible for polyhydramnios?

d] What are the possible complications of polyhydramnios?

e] Which view should be taken to document polyhydramnios?

91 a] What are some of the effects of premature rupture of the membranes (PROM) on the fetus.

b] What is the role of ultrasound in the management of these cases?

92 a] In which clinical conditions can oligohydramnios be seen on ultrasound?

b] What are some of the causes of oligo- and anhydramnios?

93 a] What is the difference in the mechanism that causes polyhydramnios in:

- CNS anomaly (e.g. meroanencephaly)
- oesophageal atresia
- the fetus of a diabetic patient.

b] Which other non-invasive tests could be done to exclude causes of polyhydramnios?

94 If you were scanning a 3rd trimester pregnancy and found polyhydramnios, which fetal structures would you check and why?

95 During an anomaly scan you could not identify the fetal stomach but saw a fairly full fetal urinary bladder. What should you do and why?

Fetal limbs

96 a] How is the fetal femur measured?

b] What factors can be responsible for obtaining an inaccurate FL measurement?

c] Which measurement will prompt you to suspect that a fetus has limb deformities (e.g. a dwarf) and how can this be excluded or confirmed?

97 In which fetal parts on ultrasound can subtle appearances be seen to suggest or confirm chromosomal abnormality?

98 a] Why is the examination of the fetal hands and feet significant?

b] Give examples of chromosomal problems which can be associated with abnormalities of the fetal hands and feet.

    c] In checking the fetal hands which points must be noted?
    d] In checking the fetal feet which points must be noted?

Chromosomal abnormalities and problems

  99 Why is it important to confirm a chromosomal abnormality in utero?

 100 a] What is the incidence of trisomy 13 (Patau's syndrome)?
      b] List the possible ultrasound findings that may suggest trisomy 13.

 101 a] What is the incidence of trisomy 18 (Edwards' syndrome)?
      b] Which ultrasound findings may suggest trisomy 18?

 102 a] What is the incidence of trisomy 21 (Down's syndrome)?
      b] Which ultrasound features may suggest trisomy 21?

 103 a] What is Turner's syndrome and what is the incidence?
      b] What ultrasound features may suggest Turner's syndrome?
      c] Which are the types of Turner's syndrome?

 104 a] What causes triploidy?
      b] Which ultrasound-identifiable structural abnormalities may be seen in fetuses with triploidy?

 105 a] What is fetal hypertelorism?
      b] How can hypertelorism be detected sonographically?
      c] What causes hypertelorism?
      d] In which conditions can hypertelorism be seen?

Fetal growth and presentation

 106 a] What is the difference between IUGR, small for dates (SFD) and SGA?
      b] Which factors influence fetal growth?
      c] Accuracy of clinical diagnosis of IUGR may be poor. Why?
      d] What makes ultrasound the best method of diagnosing IUGR?

 107 Which ultrasound-recognizable features may be responsible for a clinical large for dates?

 108 Which ultrasound-recognizable features may be responsible for a clinical small for dates?

 109 a] List the types of IUGR.
      b] Why is it important to examine in detail the anatomy in an IUGR fetus?
      c] Why is it important that IUGR be diagnosed in utero?
      d] List the causes and problems associated with each type of IUGR.
      e] Which ultrasound management may be adopted for symmetrical IUGR?
      f] Which ultrasound management may be adopted for asymmetrical IUGR?
      g] Which provisions should, if possible, be made by the ultrasound department in monitoring IUGR fetuses and why?
      h] How often should a suspected or confirmed IUGR fetus be scanned and why?

 110 Describe the parameters of the biophysical profile.

111 What is the difference between fetal tone and fetal movement?

112 When is the best time to assess a growth-retarded fetus and why?

113 How best can the growth of a fetus be assessed and which other information may be gained?

114 a] Which ultrasound-recognizable conditions can be responsible for breech or transverse fetal presentation in late pregnancy?

    b] In breech or transverse fetal presentation what other measurement should the sonographer report and why?

    c] In a fetus presenting as breech in the late 3rd trimester, which other information should the sonographer record and why?

115 a] For which clinical conditions may an ultrasound estimate of fetal weight be requested?

    b] Which two sets of parameters can be used in ultrasound fetal weight estimation and what is the advantage of not using the BPD?

Maternal problems in pregnancy

116 Why do women with pregnancy-induced high blood pressure (HBP) need serial ultrasound scans?

117 Babies born to insulin-dependent mothers are prone to which ultrasound-recognizable conditions?

118 Why is it important for pregnant diabetic patients to have serial ultrasound scans?

119 a] The following patients were referred for anomaly scan. What particular factors should the sonographer bear in mind in performing their scans and interpreting their scan findings – and why?:

    — lady with poorly controlled insulin-dependent diabetes

    — lady on cocaine

    — lady on warfarin derivatives

    — lady on lithium

    — lady on diazepam

    — lady who is a dwarf

    — lady on anticonvulsant medication

    — lady who is a chronic alcoholic.

    b] The following patients were referred for growth scan early in the 3rd trimester. What particular factors should the sonographer bear in mind in performing their scans and interpreting their scan findings – and why?:

    — lady who suffers from systemic lupus erythematosus (SLE)

    — lady who suffers from uncontrolled sickle cell disease

    — lady who is a heavy cigarette smoker (≥ 20 a day)

    — lady who is known HIV +ve.

    — lady with pre-eclampsia

    — lady with poorly controlled insulin-dependent diabetes

    — lady on cocaine.

Multiple pregnancy

120 a] Which type of twin is more prone to congenital abnormality?
- b] How often may women with multiple pregnancy require a serial ultrasound scan?
- c] Multiple pregnancy is prone to which ultrasound-recognizable problems?
- d] What is the twin–twin transfusion syndrome (TTTS)?
- e] Which ultrasound features best confirm a conjoined twin?
- f] Which factors influence perinatal survival of conjoined twins?
- g] What is the stuck twin syndrome?

121 What is an acardiac acephalic monster?

122 What are some of the fetal risks associated with multiple gestation?

123 What are some of the maternal risks associated with multiple gestation?

124 What are the major congenital abnormalities associated with MZ twins?

125 What are some of the ultrasound-recognizable conditions that may affect twins in utero?

126 What can polyhydramnios cause in twin pregnancy?

127 What is the incidence of the death of one twin from the 2nd trimester?

128 Why is serial ultrasound recommended for multiple pregnancies especially in the late 2nd and 3rd trimester?

Others

129 a] List the possible ultrasound findings that confirm IUD in the 2nd or 3rd trimester.
- b] What are some of the causes of IUD in the 2nd or 3rd trimester?

130 What are some of the risks associated with pregnancies and with children of heavy cigarette smokers (e.g. ≥ 20 cigarettes per day)?

The fetal heart

131 In a normal fetal heart describe the following:
- aorta
- crux
- foramen ovale
- interatrial septum
- interventricular septum
- mitral valve
- moderator band
- pulmonary veins
- tricuspid valve.

132 Describe the ultrasound position of the normal fetal heart in a 4-chamber (4C) plane.

133 What are the ultrasound features of a normal and acceptable 2nd trimester 4C plane?

134 What are some of the causes of the fetal heart deviating from this position?

135 What are the differences and similarities of the pulmonary artery (PA) and the aorta (Ao)?

136 a] Which ultrasound features should make the sonographer suspicious of an abnormal heart size or chest size?

b] How may a congenital abnormality of the fetal heart present on ultrasound?

c] Which clinical conditions may be suggested by fetal cardiac enlargement?

137 What could make one or more chambers of the fetal heart larger or smaller than normal?

138 In which clinical conditions are the following chambers larger than normal: RV, RA, LV, LA?

139 In which clinical conditions are the following chambers smaller than normal: RV, LV?

140 In which clinical conditions could the following be seen?:
— small PA
— small aorta
— large aorta.

141 a] What is fetal tachycardia?

b] What is the clinical significance of fetal tachycardia?

142 What is fetal bradycardia?

143 What is the clinical significance of an irregular heart rhythm in fetuses 30 weeks or more GA?

144 When should referral to a specialized fetal cardiologist be considered with respect to suspicious fetal heart rhythms?

145 In a normal fetal heart, describe what the LVOT demonstrates.

146 In a normal fetal heart, describe what the right ventricular outflow tract (RVOT) demonstrates.

147 In a normal fetal heart at about 20 weeks, describe what the transverse arches plane demonstrates from the left to the right.

148 Why is it important to assess the ventricular septum?

149 a] What is an atrioventricular septal defect (AVSD)?

b] What is a ventricular septal defect (VSD)?

150 Which ultrasound features could help to confirm a small pericardial effusion on the 4C plane?

151 What is the clinical significance of pericardial effusion?

152 What are some of the causes of pericardial effusion?

153 Images from a normal fetus are illustrated in Fig. 5.153a–c.

a] Identify the views in Fig. 5.153a–c.

b] In Fig. 5.153a identify the fetal sides and indicate what makes you sure of this.

c] Identify the structures labelled i–v in Fig. 5.153a.

d] In Fig. 5.153b identify:
— the chambers of the heart (RV, RA, LV, LA)
— the TV offsetting/hinge point
— crux

— FO
— IAS
— IVS
— Dao
— spine
— rib.

e] In Fig. 5.153c identify the structures labelled i–vii.

5.153a

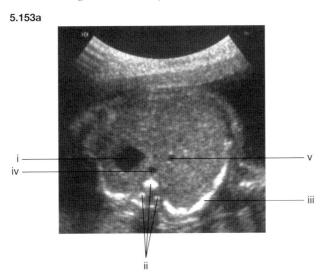

5.153b

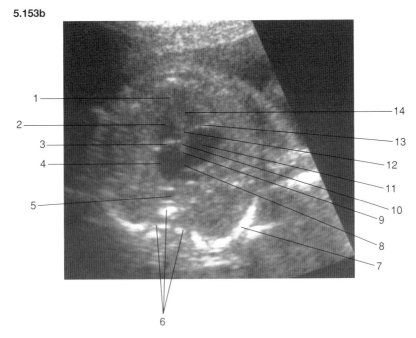

5.153c

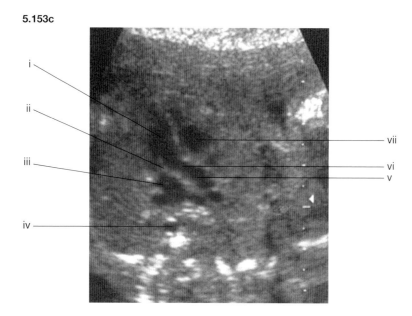

Case presentations

154 Lady C has been referred for her first scan in your department, having recently moved into the area. LMP is unknown. Going by the EDD from a previous scan in another hospital, she should be 29/40. However, by your ultrasound measurements, the fetus is 25 + 4/40.

a] What may cause this discrepancy?

b] How should you approach interpreting these scan findings and why?

155 Ladies J and K, each with a singleton pregnancy, had an anomaly scan at 20/40. Below are the fetal head ultrasound measurements in mm:

Patient	BPD	HC	AVHR	PVHR	TCD
Lady J	48	175	8/23	11/23	20
Lady K	43	175	9/21	12/21	20

a] How should you interpret the ventricular measurements in the fetuses?

b] How may ultrasound be used in the future management of these pregnancies?

6.9a

6.9b Left.

6.9c

6.9d Right.

6.9e

6.9f Left.

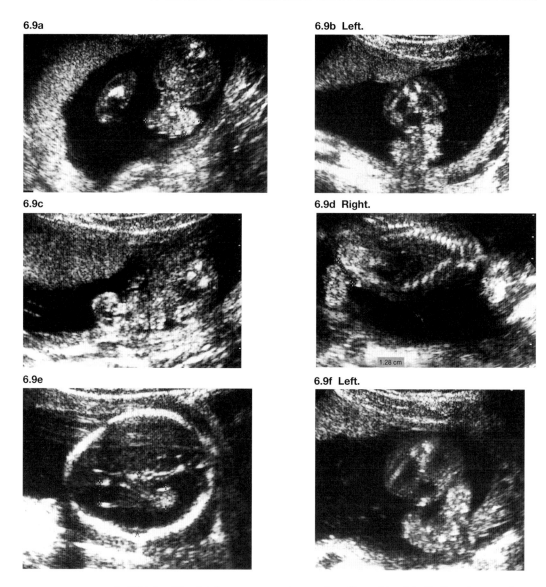

1.28 cm

e] Which of the fetal measurements may be affected by this finding, how and why?

f] What is the role of ultrasound in the future management of this pregnancy?

10. This lady was referred for a scan in the 2nd trimester with a history of loin pain. A single fetus was seen with fetal heartbeat (FHB) and movements. Fetal measurements were equal to dates. Fig. 6.10 illustrates the other maternal findings.

a] Describe the ultrasound findings and identify the condition.

b] How can ultrasound be useful in the future management of this pregnancy?

6.9g

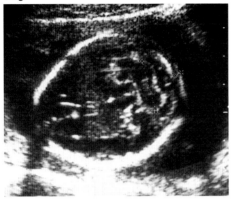

11. This lady was referred for anomaly scan. Fig. 6.11 illustrates the ultrasound findings. Fetal measurements were equal to dates.
    a] Identify the structures labelled a–h in Fig. 6.11a–c.
    b] Describe the ultrasound appearances.
    c] Should the sonographer measure the entity in Fig. 6.11a, and why or why not?
    d] Approximately how old was this fetus at the time of the scan and how did you arrive at this GA?

6.10a

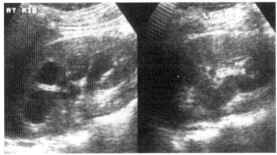

6.10b

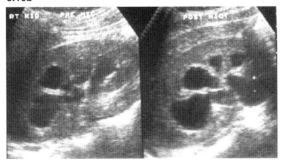

6.10c Right postmicturition.

6.10d

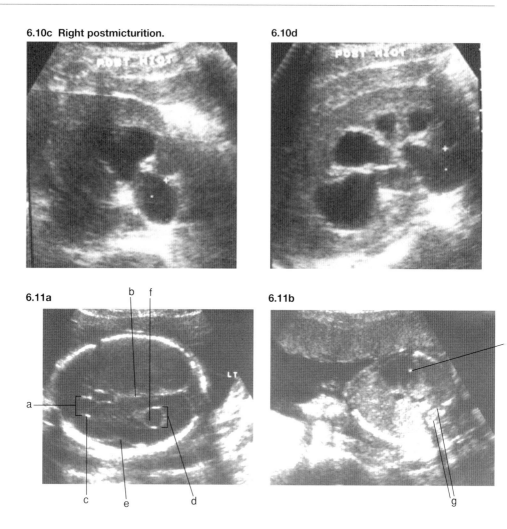

6.11a

b f

a

c e d

6.11b

g

6.11c + = 1.99 cm

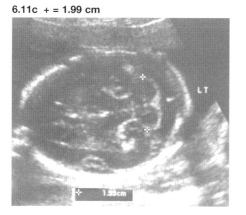

e] What is the role of ultrasound in the present and future management of this pregnancy?

12 This lady in her early thirties was referred for growth scan at 28/40. FHB and movements were seen. Fetal measurements were equal to dates. No history of per vagina (PV) bleed. Fig. 6.12 shows the other ultrasound findings.

a] Describe the ultrasound appearances.

b] What is the differential diagnosis?

c] Should the sonographer measure these entities? Why or why not?

d] What is the role of ultrasound in the present and future management of this pregnancy?

13. Fig. 6.13 illustrates the findings of a routine anomaly scan in a lady who was in her twenties.

a] Describe the ultrasound appearances.

b] What is the diagnosis and how can this be confirmed?

c] What other fetal structures should the sonographer note in the scan report and why?

6.12a ++ = 94.1 × 64.6 × 70.7 mm.   **6.12b**

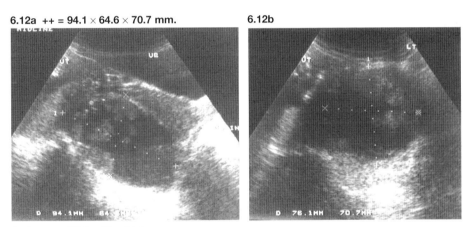

6.12c ++ = 52.3 × 31 × 21.6 mm.

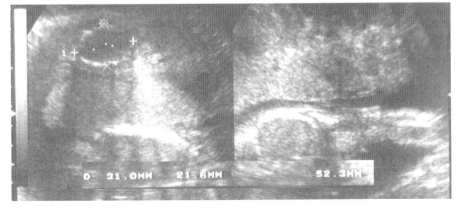

6.13a

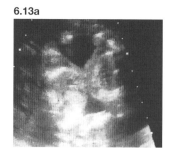

6.13b

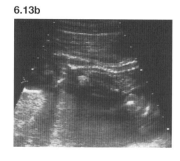

6.13c Transverse section.

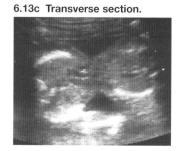

d] What is the role of ultrasound in the present and future management of this pregnancy?

e] How may this finding affect future management of this pregnancy?

14. This lady in her early thirties was referred for an emergency scan following spontaneous rupture of the membranes (SROM). Previous medical history – primary infertility, conceived through in vitro fertilization (IVF). Fig. 6.14 illustrates the ultrasound findings. Fetal measurements were: BPD = 43 mm = 18^{+6}; HC = 160 mm = 19^{+0}; FL = 21 mm = 16^{+0}; AC = unobtainable.

a] Describe the ultrasound appearances.

b] What is the diagnosis and which ultrasound findings help to confirm this?

6.14a

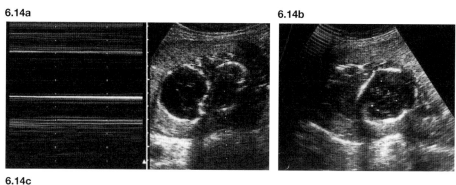

6.14b

6.14c

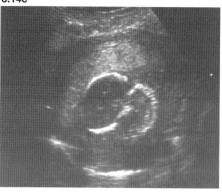

6.15a

6.15b

6.15c

6.15d Amniotic fluid surrounding twin 2.

6.15e

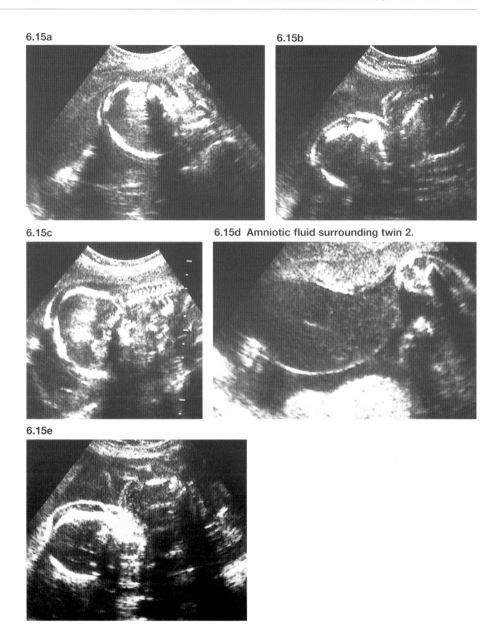

    c] Which technical problems may be encountered in performing this scan?

    d] What was the role of ultrasound in this patient?

15. Routine growth scan at 26 weeks for these twins revealed the following ultrasound appearance of twin 2 and the measurements of both twins. Previous anomaly scan revealed no obvious fetal abnormality in the twins. Two sacs, two placentas – anterior and posterior – were noted. FHB and movements were noted in twin 1.

6.17e

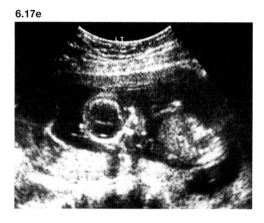

d] What is the role of ultrasound in the present and future management of this pregnancy?

18 Fig. 6.18 illustrates the findings of a routine anomaly scan. Fetal measurements were equal to dates and both lower limbs had the same appearance.

a] Identify the structures labelled a–e in Fig. 6.18.

b] Describe the fetal feet position.

c] Name this condition and list the possible causes.

d] What is the significance of this finding?

19 Fig. 6.19 illustrates findings noted during an anomaly scan.

a] Describe the ultrasound findings.

b] Name this condition.

c] Will the movements of this fetus be restricted in utero? Why or why not?

6.18

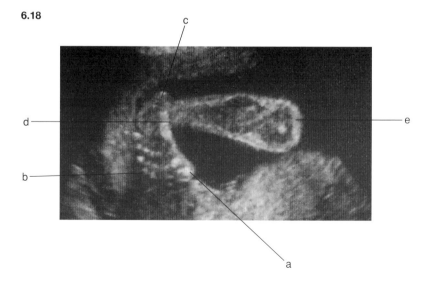

6.19a

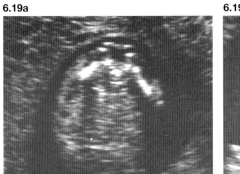

6.19b

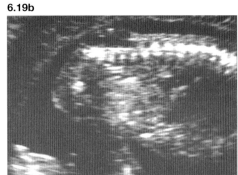

6.19c

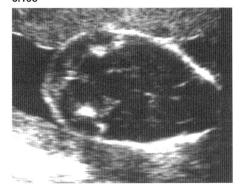

20. Fig. 6.20 illustrates the findings of an anomaly scan.
    a] Describe the ultrasound findings.
    b] Name this condition and define the incidence.
    c] Where else should the sonographer check and why?

6.20

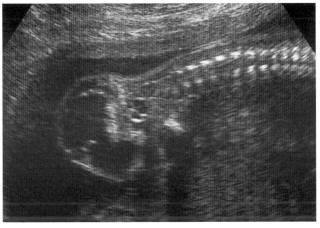

6.34c

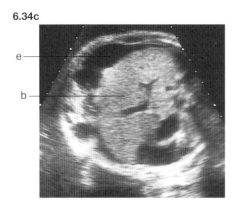

6.34d

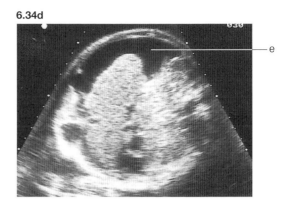

a] Identify the structures labelled a–e in Fig. 6.34a–d.

b] Describe the ultrasound findings.

c] How may these findings affect the fetus and why?

d] In which ways could ultrasound be useful in the future management of this pregnancy?

35 Fig. 6.35 illustrates the findings of a 2nd trimester scan.

a] Describe the ultrasound findings.

b] What is the possible diagnosis?

c] Where else should the sonographer check and why?

36 Fig. 6.36 illustrates the findings of a 2nd trimester scan.

a] Identify the structures labelled a–d in Fig. 6.36a–b.

b] Describe the ultrasound findings.

c] What can cause the findings in Fig. 6.36a?

d] How can ultrasound be useful in any subsequent pregnancy in this lady?

37 Fig. 6.37 illustrates the findings of a 3rd trimester scan.

a] Identify structures a–c in Fig. 6.37.

b] Describe the ultrasound findings.

6.35a

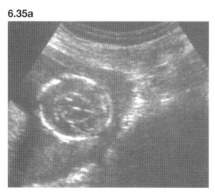

6.35b

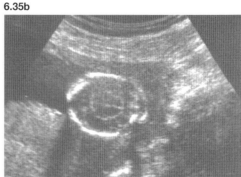

6.36a   6.36b

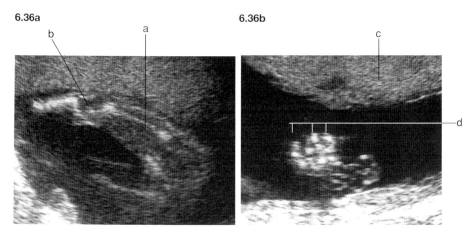

38 Fig. 6.38 illustrates the findings of an anomaly scan.
   a] Describe the ultrasound appearance of the thoracic cage.
   b] What is the clinical significance of this finding?
   c] How can ultrasound be useful in the present and future management of this pregnancy?

6.37a   6.37b

6.37c   6.37d

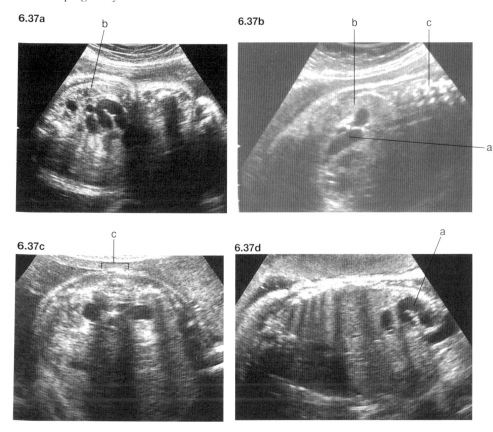

58 This lady was scanned at 24 + 3/40. Fetal measurements were equal to dates. The ultrasound appearance in Fig. 6.58 persisted throughout the scan.
   a] Describe the ultrasound findings.
   b] What is the possible condition?
   c] What is the clinical significance of this finding?
   d] How else could this patient be assessed with ultrasound?

59 Fig. 6.59 illustrates the findings of a scan at 20/40.
   a] Describe the ultrasound findings.
   b] What is the clinical significance of this finding?

60 Fig. 6.60 illustrates a transverse section of a fetus at the level of the liver at 21/40.
   a] Describe the ultrasound findings.
   b] What is the role of ultrasound in the future management of this pregnancy?

61 Fig. 6.61 illustrates the findings of an anomaly scan at 20/40.
   a] What is the cystic area posterior to the cerebellum?
   b] Is this cystic area of clinical significance?

62 Fig. 6.62 illustrates the findings of an anomaly scan.
   a] Identify the structures i–iv in Fig. 6.62a–b.
   b] What view is this?
   c] Describe the ultrasound appearances.
   d] What condition is this?
   e] Is this finding of any clinical significance?

6.60

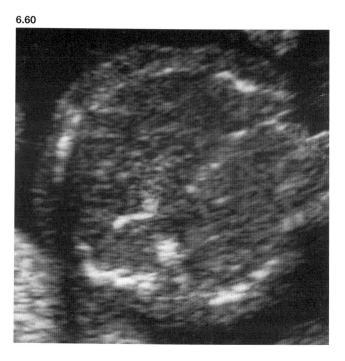

6.61

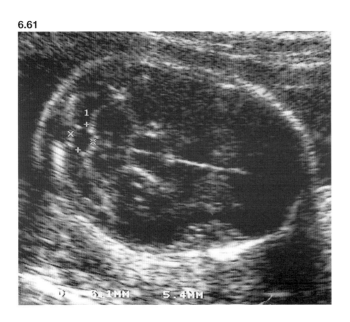

6.62a   **6.62b**

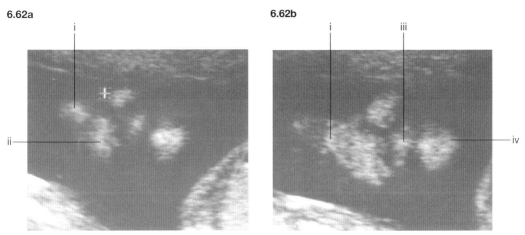

63 This lady was scanned at 24 + 6/40 with a history of IUGR.
a] What are the following indices of measurement: PI, RI, S/D ratio?
b] What do these waveforms suggest?
c] In which way could ultrasound be useful in the future management of this pregnancy?

64 A 2nd trimester scan revealed the kidney illustrated in Fig. 6.64.
a] Describe the ultrasound appearance.
b] What condition can this be?
c] Can this finding affect the urinary bladder and, if so, in which way?

6.78a ++ 62.4 mm.

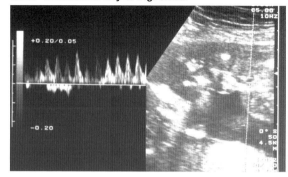

6.78b Umbilical artery to Fig. 6.78a.

6.79a ++ 28.8 mm.

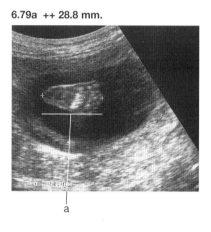

6.79b

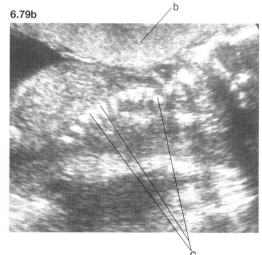

6.79c

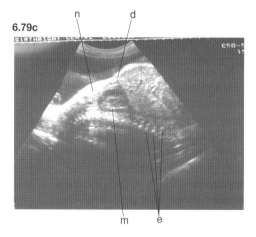

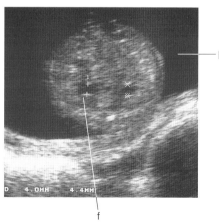

6.79e

6.79f **D = 12.3 mm × 13.0 mm**

6.79g **D = 16.3 mm.**

6.79h

6.79i **D = 15.4 mm.**

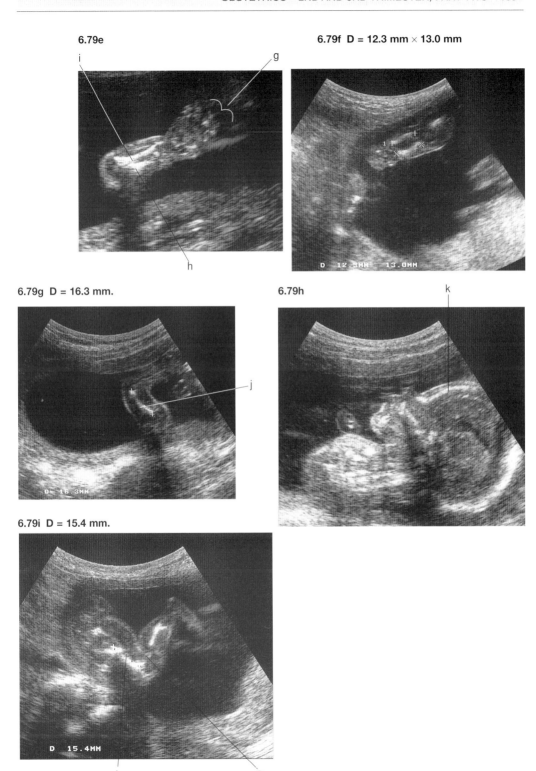

79 The fetus illustrated in Fig. 6.79 was scanned at 19/40.
   a] Identify the structures labelled a–p in Fig. 6.79.
   b] Describe the ultrasound findings.
   c] What is the likely condition?
   d] In which way can ultrasound be useful in the future management of this pregnancy?

80 Fig. 6.80a illustrates the ultrasound findings at 22/40. The karyotype was normal and no other obvious structural abnormality was seen. Fig. 6.80b and 6.80c illustrate the findings 3 weeks later.
   a] Describe the ultrasound findings.
   b] What is the likely condition?
   c] What can cause this finding?

81 Fig. 6.81 illustrates the findings of a 2nd trimester scan.
   a] Describe the shape of the fetal head.
   b] What is the clinical significance of this finding?

6.80a 9.8 mm, 24.4 mm, 11.7 mm.

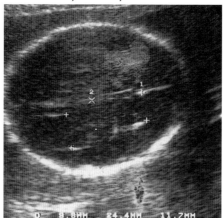

6.80b

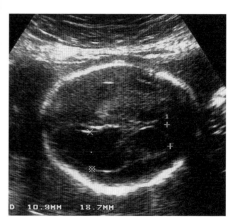

6.80c

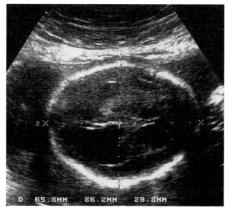

6.81

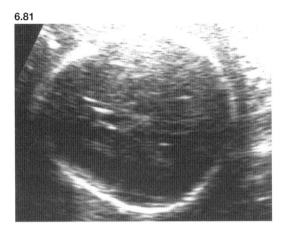

6.82a TS abdomen.

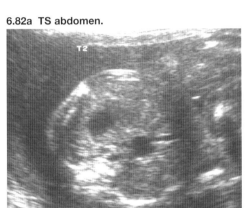

6.82b

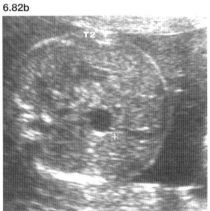

82 Fig. 6.82 illustrates the findings of an anomaly scan at 22/40.
  a] Describe the ultrasound appearance.
  b] What could this be?
  c] How else could the condition be confirmed?

83 Fig. 6.83 illustrates ultrasound findings at 20/40. Fetal karyotype was normal.
  a] Identify the structures labelled i–vii in Fig. 6.83a–c.
  b] Describe the ultrasound findings.
  c] How can ultrasound be useful in the future management of this pregnancy?

84 Fig. 6.84 illustrates ultrasound findings at 16/40.
  a] How best can the kidney echo pattern be determined?
  b] Describe the ultrasound findings.
  c] What else should be mentioned in the scan report?
  d] What is the clinical significance of these findings?
  e] How can ultrasound be useful in the future management of this pregnancy?

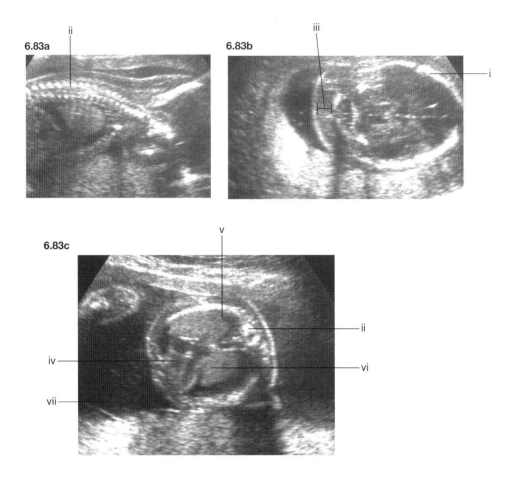

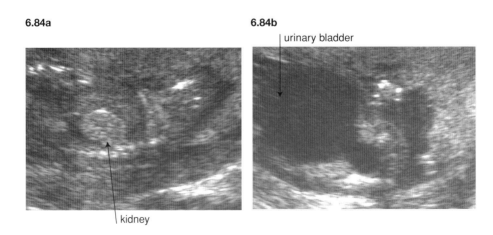

6.85

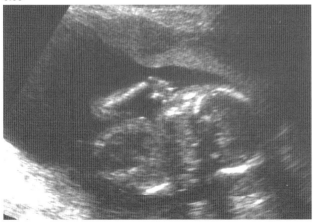

85 Fig. 6.85 illustrates ultrasound findings during a scan. This limb was noted to be in the same position throughout the examination and during subsequent scans.
  a] Describe the ultrasound findings of this upper limb.
  b] What can this be?
  c] What else should the sonographer check and why?
  d] What is the clinical significance of this finding?
86 A scan at 15/40 revealed the fetal head illustrated in Fig. 6.86.
  a] Describe the ultrasound finding.
  b] What could this be?
  c] Which of the fetal measurements is likely to be affected by this finding?
  d] Which of these will detect this lesion and why – MSAFP or ultrasound?
  e] What is the clinical significance of this finding?
  f] Which other diagnostic tests may be required in this instance and why?

6.86

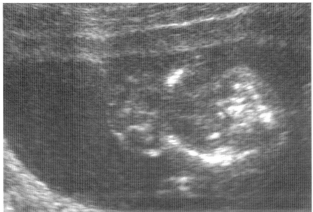

6.87

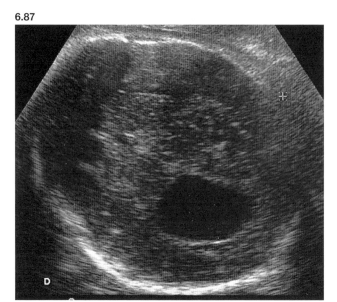

87 Fig. 6.87 illustrates ultrasound findings at 33/40.
   a] Describe the ultrasound findings.
   b] What could this be?
   c] How can one be sure of the entity?
   d] What else should the sonographer mention in the scan report?
   e] In which way could ultrasound be useful in the future management of this pregnancy?

88 Fig. 6.88 illustrates the findings of an anomaly scan.
   a] Describe the ultrasound finding.
   b] What is the clinical significance of this finding?

6.88

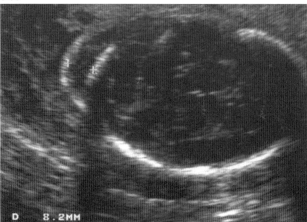

89 This fetus was scanned at 16/40. Fig. 6.89 illustrates the ultrasound findings.
   a] Identify the sections in Fig. 6.89d and e and the structures labelled 1 and 2.
   b] Describe the significant ultrasound findings in Fig. 6.89a–e.
   c] What are the likely conditions demonstrated?
90 Fig. 6.90 illustrates ultrasound findings at 38/40.
   a] Describe the ultrasound findings.
   b] What is the possible condition?
   c] What is the clinical significance of these findings?

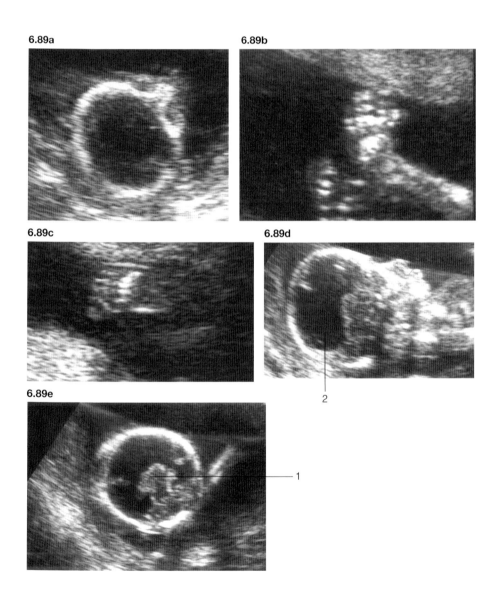

6.89a

6.89b

6.89c

6.89d

2

6.89e

1

6.103g

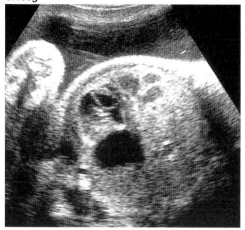

6.103h Some days later.

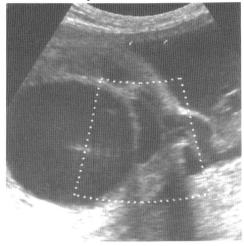

6.103i Some days later.

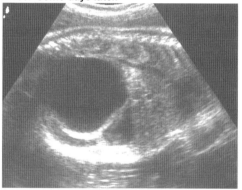

6.103j Some days later.

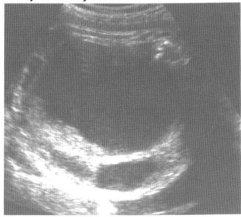

6.103k 1.4 × 64.9 × 67.4 mm. Some days later.

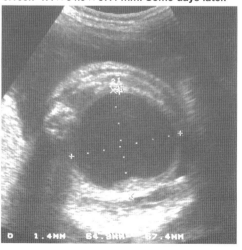

Fertility

LEARNING OBJECTIVES

By the end of working through this chapter the reader should:

- know some of the causes of female infertility
- know why a baseline gynaecological scan prior to fertility treatment is essential
- be aware of congenital uterine anomalies and the implication on fertility
- know the conditions that a sonographer needs to fulfil during monthly fertility treatment scanning
- be aware of the role of ultrasound during a monitored or treatment cycle
- know what follicles are
- be aware of what anovulation is and the possible ultrasound features
- be aware of amenorrhoea, its types and causes
- be aware of what ovarian hyperstimulation syndrome (OHSS) is, the types and the use of ultrasound in identifying and managing OHSS
- be aware of some causes of subfertility in a couple, some of the fertility treatment options available in the UK and some of the possible factors influencing a couple's choice of fertility treatment
- be aware of some common medical terminology
- be aware of some tests for the investigation of female infertility
- know what hyperprolactinaemia is
- understand short and long in vitro fertilization protocols
- be familiar with uterine cavity and tubal assessment
- be aware of leiomyoma and how it may affect fertility
- appreciate the role of ultrasound following a successful or an unsuccessful treatment cycle
- be aware of the incidence and implications of an ectopic pregnancy with fertility treatment
- understand the role of ultrasound in postcoital testing
- know what a luteal phase defect is
- understand polycystic ovary (PCO) and polycystic ovarian disease (PCOD) and their differences
- know what a chemical pregnancy is
- in each case presented be able to:
  —identify normal and abnormal ultrasound patterns in the images
  —write an ultrasound report from the images
  —suggest the possible condition/alternatives
  —suggest which organs/structures should be checked and why
  —understand the implications of the demonstrated conditions
  —be aware of the ultrasound role in the management of the case presented
  —be informed of the presented case outcome where known.

INTRODUCTION

Approximately 1 in 6 couples will experience fertility problems at some time in their reproductive lives. Infertility has been defined as an involuntary failure to conceive within 12 months of unprotected intercourse. It has been observed that approximately 90% of couples with normal fertility will conceive in the first year, while 95% will have conceived within 2 years, with the chances of conception decreasing with time after this 2-year period.

There are about 100 clinics spread throughout the UK which offer in vitro fertilization (IVF) treatment, either free under the NHS or in private units within or outside NHS premises. Many factors have made fertility treatment more available and sonographers are being involved as part of the fertility team in specialized units or district general hospitals.

Many of the couples classified as subfertile live normal, busy lives. However, subfertility is often accompanied by high levels of anxiety and emotional distress which may affect the individuals and society in general. The sonographer should be aware of their organization's protocol in communicating the ultrasound findings. While many patients would like to be shown the television screen and talked through the findings, for various reasons some may prefer not to be shown. Cultural differences may also affect the presence or absence of the husband or partner during a scan. For example, it has been observed that many ladies of Eastern origin find it too embarrassing to have their husband in for their scan.

By the time a couple get referred to a specialized fertility unit, either by self-referral or by their GP, they may have already been through some form of fertility treatment which has not worked. As a result of this, however, they may be aware of terms like follicles, hyperstimulation, etc.

Fertility treatment could be a stressful time for the couple. The sonographer should be aware of some of the fears experienced and sometimes expressed by the patients such as:

- At the initial consultation scan: *What will they find? Will the scan reveal something that will make me unsuitable for the treatment?*
- During treatment scans: *Are my eggs growing? Am I responding to the treatment as expected? Will my treatment be stopped?*
- First scan after a positive pregnancy test: *Does the baby look OK? Is it in the right place? Is there any heartbeat? How many babies are there?*
- First scan after a failed fertility treatment: *What went wrong? Will my treatment ever be successful?*

Sonographers are not counsellors but will need to apply appropriate counselling skills, and should be compassionate and supportive. Flexibility is essential in making scan appointments for the patients because of conflicting social and work roles.

Fertility treatment may equally be stressful for the sonographer for many reasons. For example, the success rate per treatment cycle in most cases is less than 50%. Ethical issues relating to the various fertility treatments provided may clash with personal beliefs. The sonographer should be aware of their organization's provision which addresses such work-related stress.

Most if not all ethical issues surrounding fertility treatment are centred around non-ultrasound related issues such as embryo storage and disposal, number of embryos to implant, reimplanting stored ovarian tissue post-therapy in order to re-establish fertility, surrogacy, genetic engineering, research on embryos, and the welfare of the unborn child resulting from fertility treatments. Sonographers need to keep up to date with current issues as patients tend to ask questions of staff in the fertility centre with the hope that they would know.

The sonographer should be familiar with the Human Fertilisation and Embryology Authority (HFEA) guidelines and the various departmental protocols regarding, for example, chaperoning during transvaginal examinations, requests for transvaginal scan (TVS) by the gynaecologist for scanning during a fertility treatment, prescan consent documentation and communicating scan results to patients.

◆ This chapter is written specifically for sonographers working in specialized fertility units.
◆ The format used and protocols referred to in this chapter in describing ultrasound appearances may differ from what is used in other units.

QUESTIONS

1 List some of the causes of female infertility that can be evaluated by ultrasound.
2 Describe the following terms as used in transvaginal ultrasound (TVS): anechoic, hyperechoic, isoechoic, hypoechoic.
3 What are some points in favour of a baseline ultrasound scan of the patient before commencing fertility treatment?
4 What is the clinical significance of congenital uterine anomalies in infertility?
5 a] Which criteria should the sonographer try to meet during a monthly infertility scanning?
  b] Why is TVS preferred for follicular monitoring rather than transabdominal (TA) scan?
6 What is the role of ultrasound during a monitored fertility cycle?
7 What is the role of ultrasound during a fertility treatment cycle?
8 For which prefertility treatment procedures could ultrasound be employed?
9 A patient is referred for a baseline scan before commencing fertility treatment. List some possible ultrasound-identifiable conditions which may be found during such a scan.
10 How do follicles appear on ultrasound?
11 In a normal unstimulated cycle what is the range of the leading follicle?
12 a] How is the corpus luteum different from the follicle on ultrasound?
  b] What is the difference between a follicle, an egg and the corpus luteum?
13 How can the hypogastric vein be differentiated from the follicle?
14 Which is smaller on ultrasound, the internal iliac vein or the internal iliac artery?
15 What are the associated risks with the use of gonadotrophins?
16 What is anovulation?
17 Which ultrasound features may be suggestive of anovulation?

18 Which ultrasound features may be suggestive of chronic anovulation?

19 Which ultrasound features may be suggestive of premature ovarian failure?

20 Which ultrasound features may be suggestive of luteinized unruptured follicle (LUF) syndrome?

21 Which ultrasound features may be suggestive of an impending ovulation?

22 Which ultrasound findings can suggest that ovulation has occurred?

23 For which fertility treatments is it important to know the time of ovulation and why?

24 What is the average growth rate of follicles?

25 List some of the factors that can affect endometrial thickness measurement.

26 What are the two types of amenorrhoea?

27 What are some of the causes of amenorrhoea?

28 What causes the ovarian hyperstimulation syndrome (OHSS)?

29 Describe the grades of OHSS.

30 Which categories of women undergoing fertility treatment are more prone to develop OHSS?

31 When does OHSS usually present?

32 How can ultrasound scanning be useful in preventing and managing OHSS?

33 What is the significance of knowing the exact time of ovulation in fertility therapies?

34 What is the significance of transmigration of the ovum?

35 A history of a normal menstrual period in a woman of child-bearing age with pelvic pain and tenderness does not rule out the possibility of an ectopic pregnancy. Why?

36 What is the 'sliding organ' sign in pelvic ultrasound?

37 What are some of the causes of subfertility in a couple?

38 List and describe the fertility treatment options currently available in the UK.

39 Describe some factors that may influence the choice of fertility treatment for a couple.

40 What do the following medical terms mean?:
    — azoospermia
    — aspermia
    — asthenozoospermia
    — teratospermia
    — normozoospermia
    — oligospermia
    — infertility
    — subfertility
    — primary infertility
    — secondary infertility.

41 Describe some tests that may be carried out in investigating a woman suffering from infertility. What might each show?

42 A woman with infertility is being investigated for hyperprolactinaemia.
    a] What is this condition?
    b] Which diagnostic tests may be requested and why?

43 a] What is the difference between short and long IVF protocols?

b] Which factors may determine the choice of protocol for a woman about to undergo IVF?

c] What are the advantages and disadvantages of these protocols?

d] Where the following protocols are used, what are the likely times for performing the ultrasound scans?

— short protocol

— ultrashort protocol

— long Day 1 protocol

— long Day 21 protocol

e] What is the possible difference between the ultrasound findings in d above?

44 Why are chorionic gonadotrophin (Profasi) or progesterone (Cyclogest) suppositories given following embyro transfer?

45 How is the LH-RH analogue meant to work in a Day 21 protocol?

46 A 34-year-old lady with primary infertility of 4 years' duration presented at the fertility clinic. She also claimed experiencing dysmenorrhoea and dyspareunia. The uterus and the right ovary had a normal echopattern but on the left was the finding illustrated in Fig. 7.46. The left ovary was not identified separately from this structure.

a] Describe this finding.

b] What is the possible ultrasound-identifiable clinical condition?

c] What is the clinical significance of this finding to fertility?

d] Which other structure may resemble this finding and how can you be sure it is not the latter.

7.46 D1 = 51.4 mm, D = 55.9 mm.

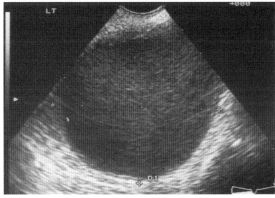

47 a] What are the types of unicornuate uterus?

b] Are there any clinical implications for unicornuate uterus?

48 Which physical and clinical conditions could make a TVS painful for the patient?

49 List the possible protective covers for the transvaginal probe.

50 Fig. 7.50 illustrates a longitudinal section of the uterus of a patient on day 10 of a stimulated gonadotrophin cycle.

7.58a

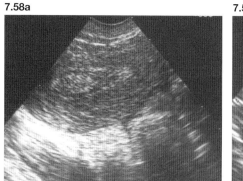

7.58b

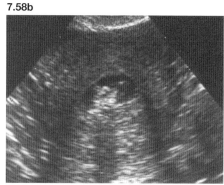

56 What is the role of ultrasound in the management of leiomyomas?

57 How may a submucous fibroid cause problems with fertility?

58 A preliminary ultrasound of the uterus of a patient intending to embark on fertility treatment revealed the finding illustrated in Fig. 7.58. Some saline was then introduced into the uterine cavity under ultrasound control.

    a] Describe the ultrasound finding in Fig. 7.58a.

    b] What was the aim in introducing some saline into the cavity?

    c] What does Fig. 7.58b demonstrate?

59 Following an unsuccessful treatment cycle what is the role of ultrasound?

60 Following a successful treatment cycle what is the role of ultrasound?

61 Fig. 7.61 illustrates the ultrasound scan findings of a patient performed on day 5 of using only the analogue nafarelin (Synarel). Some fluid was also seen in the POD.

    a] Describe the ultrasound findings.

    b] What is the possible reason for such findings?

7.61a

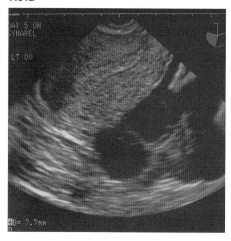

7.61b

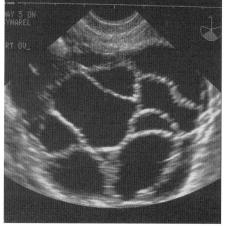

7.62

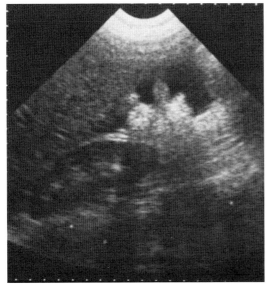

62 Following egg collection and embryo transfer, a patient returned some days later
     with complaints of abdominal distension, nausea, shortness of breath and
     vomiting. An abdominal scan was requested. Fig. 7.62 illustrates a longitudinal
     section of the right upper quadrant.
     a] Describe the ultrasound findings.
     b] Which other possible ultrasound appearances can one expect to find in the pelvis?
     c] Name this condition.

7.63

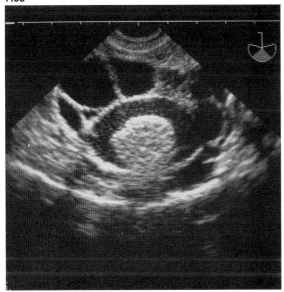

63 Fig. 7.63 illustrates an ultrasound of an ovary of a 25-year-old lady.
a] Describe the ultrasound appearance.
b] Which possible entity can this be?
c] How can this affect the patient's fertility?

64 An initial consultation scan of a patient seeking fertility treatment revealed the finding illustrated in Fig. 7.64. Both ovaries and the uterus had a normal ultrasound appearance. Ultrasound findings were from the RIF.
a] Describe this finding.
b] What is the most likely condition demonstrated in Fig. 7.64?
c] How may this affect the success of fertility?
d] What are the possible options for managing this finding?

65 This lady was referred for a pretreatment baseline scan. The uterus and the left ovary had a normal echopattern. On the right were the findings illustrated in Fig. 7.65. The right ovary was not seen separate from the structure in Fig. 7.65b.
a] Describe the ultrasound appearances in Fig. 7.65a.
b] Describe the ultrasound appearances in Fig. 7.65b.

66 An initial consultation ultrasound scan of a patient revealed the ovarian appearance illustrated in Fig. 7.66.
a] Describe this finding.
b] What is the most likely condition demonstrated in Fig. 7.66?
c] How may this affect her fertility?
d] What are the possible ultrasound-recognizable responses to fertility drugs which may be seen in such a patient?

67 Three weeks after a positive pregnancy test following fertility treatment, no intrauterine pregnancy was demonstrated on the ultrasound. Fig. 7.67 illustrates the only significant ultrasound finding.
a] Describe this finding.
b] What is the most likely condition demonstrated in Fig. 7.67?

7.64 +D = 120 mm, XD = 77 mm.

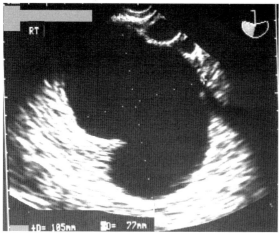

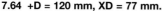

7.65a +D = 120 mm.

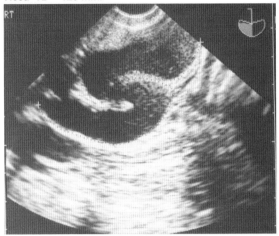

7.65b +D = 27 mm, XD = 45 mm.

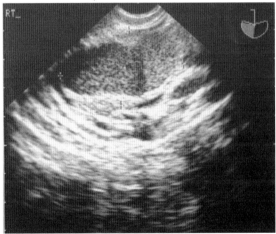

68 a] Which group of patients is prone to ectopic pregnancy?
  b] What is a heterotopic pregnancy?
  c] What is the incidence of heterotopic pregnancy?
  d] List some of the possible clinical presentations of an ectopic pregnancy.
69 A 28-year-old woman with a known very irregular menstrual cycle was referred for an initial consultation scan at a fertility unit on 18 June 1995. The patient claimed she usually has, on average, two menstrual periods in a year. Her known last menstrual period was 4 February 1995. Both ovarian echopattern and size appeared normal on ultrasound. Fig. 7.69 illustrates the other ultrasound findings.
  a] Describe the ultrasound finding in Fig. 7.69a.
  b] Which ultrasound image displays are demonstrated in Fig. 7.69b?
  c] What is the ultrasound finding in this patient?

7.66

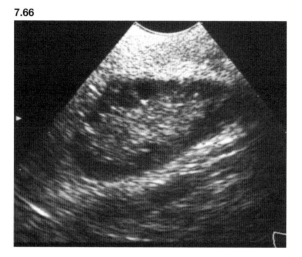

7.67 +D = 2.4 mm.

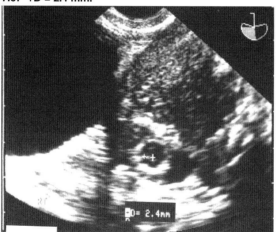

d] Do the ultrasound findings correlate with the patient's dates. If not, what could have been responsible for this?

70 Thickening of the endometrium cannot be used as a means of diagnosing pregnancy. Why?

71 This lady undergoing fertility treatment started analogue on day 21 of her cycle. She has a 28–30-day regular cycle. However, 19 days later her period had not started. A pregnancy test was negative. Fig. 7.71 illustrates the ultrasound findings.

a] Describe the ultrasound findings.

b] What is the possible ultrasound finding which might have been the cause of this patient not menstruating as expected?

7.69a +D = 12 mm.

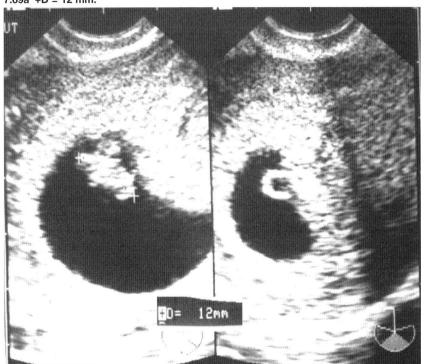

7.69b

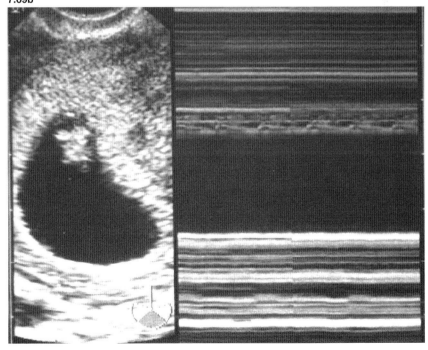

7.71a

7.71b

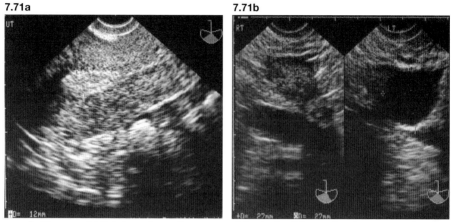

c] How could this have been the cause of the lack of the patient's menstrual period?

72 Why is a Day 3 scan requested in a patient undergoing fertility treatment on a long Day 21 protocol?

73 What is the use of ultrasound in the postcoital test?

74 Following fertility treatment, a lady became pregnant. Fig. 7.74 illustrates the ultrasound findings at 7 + 4/40. No FHB was seen in sac 2.

7.74 +D = 13 mm, XD = 3.6 mm.

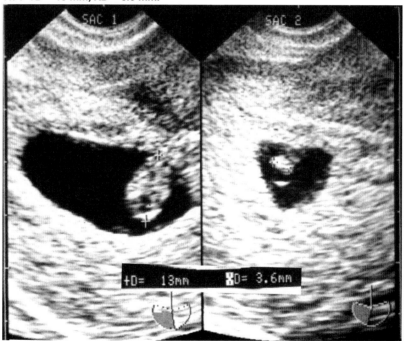

a] Describe the ultrasound appearances.

b] What conclusions can be made from the ultrasound images?

75 Fig. 7.75 illustrates a uterus ultrasound scan at 5 + 4/40 following fertility treatment.

a] Describe the ultrasound findings.

b] What are some of the associated risks in multiple pregnancy?

76 Fig. 7.76 illustrates a uterus ultrasound scan at 5/40 following fertility treatment. Describe the ultrasound findings.

77 Following IVF treatment, a patient became pregnant. Fig. 7.77 illustrates the longitudinal section of the uterus at 5/40 GA. FHB was present (not demonstrated here).

a] Describe the ultrasound appearances.

b] What could the echopoor area next to the gestational sac represent?

c] How best could the echopoor area be assessed?

7.75 +D = 13 mm, XD = 15 mm.

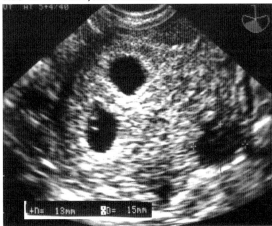

7.76

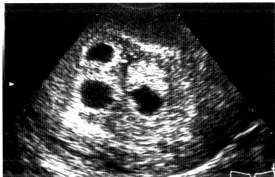

Anatomy

ANSWERS

1 a] Shaped like an inverted pear, the normal uterus is divided into the fundus, body and cervix (Fig. A1.1a). The fundus is the dome-shaped roof of the uterus, located between the two uterine tubes; it also acts as the sac for gestation. The isthmus, which is about 10 mm in length, is the narrow region between the body and the cervix and develops during the later part of the pregnancy. The cervix, which opens into the vagina, is narrow and acts as sphincter during pregnancy. The cervix is the strong pivotal point for uterine stability, being attached to the pelvic walls by the pubocervical ligament anteriorly, uterosacral posteriorly and transverse cervical laterally. The uterus is supported by the broad, uterosacral, cardinal and round ligaments.

Blood supply is by the uterine arteries, a branch of the internal iliac artery and the arcuate arteries. Venous drainage is via the uterine veins.

Nerve supply is via the sympathetic and parasympathetic nerves.

b] The uterus develops in utero from the two mullerian ducts. Development starts at 3–4/40 and continues into the 2nd trimester. Interruption to this process causes incomplete fusion.

Common uterine abnormalities include:
— failure of the uterus to mature at puberty, thus retaining its infantile form
— unicornuate uterus and absence of the uterine tube on the other side due to the absence of one paramesonephric duct during development (Fig. A1.1b)
— bicornuate uterus, consisting of double uterine cavities separated by a septum (Fig. A1.1c)
— uterus duplex, otherwise called uterus didelphys, where there are two separate uteri, each connected to a uterine tube and each possessing its own cervical opening; there may also be a double vagina (Fig. A1.1d)
— uterus subseptus, comprising two vaginas, two cervices and two uterine cavities but only a single medial wall (Fig. A1.1e).

A1.1a–e

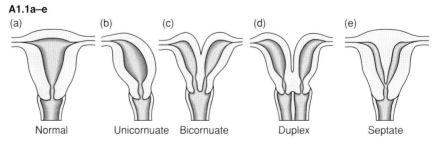

(a) Normal (b) Unicornuate (c) Bicornuate (d) Duplex (e) Septate

- ◆ Uterine abnormalities are often associated with premature labour and spontaneous abortion.
- ◆ Uterine structural defects are seen in 1–2% of the female population and cause recurrent abortions rather than failure to conceive.

2 The uterus:
— is the site of menstruation
— provides a pathway for the sperm to reach the uterine tubes
— is the site of fertilized ovum implantation
— is the site for fetal development during pregnancy
— is the site for labour.
The lower cervix has the multiple function of being a passageway, a barrier and a reservoir at different times.

3 The uterus lies posterior to the bladder, cephalad to the vagina and anterior to the rectum. It is usually anteverted but is sometimes retroverted; in the midline it may be lightly rotated to the right or left.

4 • Internal os: where the isthmus joins the cervical canal
  • External os: where the cervix opens into the vagina
  • Endometrium: inner layer of the uterus. It is very vascular, made up of ciliated and secretory cells, endometrial glands and connective tissue. The endometrium gets shed in the menstrual period. It is also the site for normal pregnancy implantation
  • Myometrium: the middle layer of the uterus and bulk of the uterine wall, it is made up of smooth muscle fibres which are thinnest at the cervix and thickest at the fundus. Coordinated muscle contractions of the myometrium help to expel the fetus during childbirth
  • Perimetrium: the outer layer of the uterus and part of the visceral peritoneum. Posteriorly, it is reflected onto the rectum forming the deep pouch of Douglas (POD), anteriorly it is reflected over the urinary bladder forming the shallow vesicouterine pouch and laterally it becomes the broad ligaments.

5 There are two ovaries which vary in size and appearance depending on the woman's age and stage in her reproductive cycle. It is suggested that in the young adult the ovary is flattened, ovoid and measures approximately $40 \times 20 \times 10$ mm. It has an upper and a lower pole and an anterior border, also referred to as the mesovarian border which forms the hilus of the ovary through which the nerves and blood vessels enter and exit. The posterior free border is convex and more rounded. Blood supply is from the ovarian arteries which arise from the aorta just below the origin of the renal arteries and from the uterine artery with a free anastomosis between these sources of blood supply. The size of the ovarian blood vessels varies depending on the functional state of the ovary and can be influenced by the gonadotrophic hormones. The left ovarian vein drains into the left renal vein and the right ovarian vein drains directly into the inferior vena cava.
Lymphatic draining follows the course of the ovarian blood vessels, with drainage into the lateral aortic and preaortic lymph nodes.
Nerve supply is via the sympathetic/parasympathetic nerve fibres.

- The lymphatics of the ovary communicate unrestrictedly with those of the uterus and the uterine tubes.
- It is unknown what determines (a) the choice of follicle that becomes dominant and ovulates and (b) whether ovulation will occur in the right or left ovary.
- Ovaries do not alternate from one cycle to another.
- The average female has about 30 years of reproductive life, releasing approximately one oocyte per ovarian cycle (about 400 oocytes in a lifetime).
- If an increased amount of gonadotrophin is administered as a fertility drug, multiple oocytes will develop in most cases.
- Removal of one ovary leads to the remaining ovary becoming larger in size by a process called *compensatory hypertrophy* (where there is a functioning pituitary gland).

6 a] During reproductive life, the ovary usually lies posterolateral to the uterus, anterior to the iliac artery and vein and medial to the ovarian vessels.
- At birth the ovaries lie high in the abdominal cavity; early in childhood they descend and come to lie below the brim of the pelvis in the ovarian fossae.
- At menopause (45–55 years), when the reproductive life of the woman ends, the cyclical changes in the ovary first become irregular and then cease altogether. The ovary gets smaller and no follicle will be seen on ultrasound.
- It is not unusual to find an ovary stuck to the uterus secondary to pelvic adhesions or sometimes high up in the pelvis, displaced by pelvic masses such as fibroids. In stimulated cycles the ovaries (as a result of increased weight) might be seen in the POD.

b] Ovarian location is affected by:
— the position of the uterus. When the uterus in pregnancy ascends into the abdominal cavity, the ovaries get pulled along and become elongated. After childbirth they return to the pelvic cavity but are now more horizontal in position
— the bowel
— the degree of urinary bladder filling
— Wertheim's surgery
— fertility treatment with multiple follicles, where it is not uncommon to find enlarged ovaries in the POD.

c] The size of the ovary depends on many factors including:
— patient's age: ovarian volume is known to be largest in 30–39 year olds and normally decreases during the menopause
— the hormonal status of the patient
— polycystic ovarian disease (PCOD), where many patients tend to have enlarged ovaries
— removal of one ovary, following which the remaining ovary may get larger (see Answer 5 above)
— fertility treatment, during which the ovaries tend to get larger due to the effect of the medication

    — ovarian hyperstimulation syndrome (OHSS) following fertility treatment, where the ovaries become larger

    — the presence of a cyst, benign neoplasm or cancer which may make the ovarian measurement larger

    — birth control pills which may affect ovarian size.

♦ It is important to be familiar with your departmental upper limit of normal measurement of the ovary.

♦ It is good practice to document ovarian measurement on each routine gynaecology ultrasound scan for easier comparison if and when necessary.

♦ An ovary that is twice the size of the other ovary is usually considered abnormal.

♦ Care should be taken not to mistake a pedunculated fibroid for an ovary.

♦ The ovary may be considered large if adjacent adhesions are mistakenly measured with the ovary.

7 The main functions of the ovary are to:

— produce a mature ovum every 28 days (for those with a 28-day regular cycle)

— secrete oestrogen and progesterone

— support pregnancy.

♦ Ovum production may take more or less time depending on the woman's cycle length.

8 a] There are two uterine tubes, one on each side of the uterus. Each uterine tube is approximately 10–12.5 cm long, pursuing a tortuous course in the free margin of the broad ligament. Tracing it laterally from the uterus, the uterine tube runs laterally in the horizontal plane to the side wall of the pelvis, then ascends in front of the ovary and arches so that the infundibulum is related to the upper part of the ovary and the fimbriae are related to its posterior and medial surface. The uterine tube is made up of the infundibulum, ampulla and isthmus.

Blood supply is from the ovarian and uterine arteries. Lymphatic supply drains mostly towards the mesovarium where it joins the ovarian vessels to form common channels ascending to the lateral and preaortic nodes. The isthmus is drained by vessels which accompany the round ligaments and reach the superficial inguinal nodes.

Nerve supply is via the sympathetic and parasympathetic nerve fibres.

b] The function of a uterine tube is to:

— convey an ovum from one of the two ovaries to the body of the uterus

— convey sperm which is deposited in the vagina during intercourse/insemination to the ovum

— provide a site for fertilization of the oocyte

— convey the zygote to the uterus.

c] The infundibulum is the funnel-shaped outer part nearest to the ovary. Its lumen communicates with the peritoneal cavity through the ostium, an opening fringed with a varying number of finger or petal-like processes known as the fimbriae. One of the fimbriae (called the *fimbriae ovarica*) is usually more prominent than the others and is attached to the posterior border or adjacent part of the inner surface of the ovary.

d] The ampulla is the widest, longest portion of the uterine tube, making up about 66% of its length.

e] The isthmus is the short, narrow, thick-walled portion of the uterine tube that joins the uterus.

- The uterine tube is influenced by sex hormones. Its muscle cells vary in size under the influence of the different ovarian phases. It is largest around the time of ovulation.
- Peristaltic movement occurs in the uterine tube but not throughout the entire length at the same time.
- The uterine tubes do not contract in harmony: each has its own rhythm, and function is dependent on peristaltic movements which diminish after ovulation.

f] A blocked tube occurs when there is an obstruction within the lumen, thus preventing it from conveying the oocyte, sperm or zygote to its desired destination. Tubal blockage may be secondary to infection or endometriosis.

g] A blocked tube can cause infertility or ectopic pregnancy.

9 a] The vagina is seen as three parallel lines posterior to the urinary bladder.

b] Haematocolpos occurs when the hymen is imperforate, resulting in trapped menstrual flow which cannot be released via the vagina.

c] The space between the vault of the vagina and the anterior lip of the cervix is referred to as the anterior fornix, the space between the posterior lip of the cervix and vagina is the posterior fornix and on each side of the cervix the vagina forms the lateral fornix. The posterior fornix is deeper than the others because of the way in which the cervix of the anteverted uterus projects backwards into the vagina.

10 (Answer in Fig. A1.10a–c on pp 206–208).

11 a] The structures in Fig. 1.11a–g comprise:

1 urinary bladder
2 uterus
3 right ovary
4 left ovary
5 vagina
6 myometrium
7 endometrium
8 fundus
9 endometrium
10 stroma
11 cervix
12 fluid in the POD
13 endometrium
14 blood vessel
15 endometrial measurement
16 corpus – body

17 isthmus

18 triple line endometrium

19 follicle.

b] Fig. 1.11a: transabdominal scan (TAS) transverse section of the uterus and ovaries

Fig. 1.11b: TAS longitudinal section of an anteverted uterus

Fig. 1.11c: transvaginal scan (TVS) longitudinal section of an anteverted uterus

Fig. 1.11d: TAS longitudinal section of a retroverted uterus

Fig. 1.11e: TAS longitudinal section of an anteverted uterus

Fig. 1.11f: TVS longitudinal section of a retroverted uterus

Fig. 1.11g: TVS longitudinal section of a retroverted uterus.

◆ The ultrasound appearance of both ovaries as seen in Fig. 1.11a is polycystic.

c] Structures 7, 9, 13 and 18 are all endometrium but in different menstrual phases. The appearance in 7 is seen early in the menstrual cycle, 9 is seen in early luteal phase, 13 in late luteal phase or early pregnancy before the gestational sac is visible and 18 is a triple line endometrium which is seen in mid-cycle.

A1.10a A median sagittal section through the female pelvis, seen from the left side.

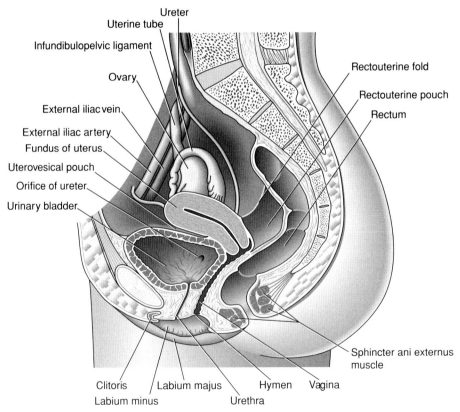

A1.10b Posterior view of the uterus, upper part of the vagina and broad ligament. The left half of the posterior wall of the uterus and of the vagina has been removed to show the appearance of the endometrium and of the vaginal mucous membrane.

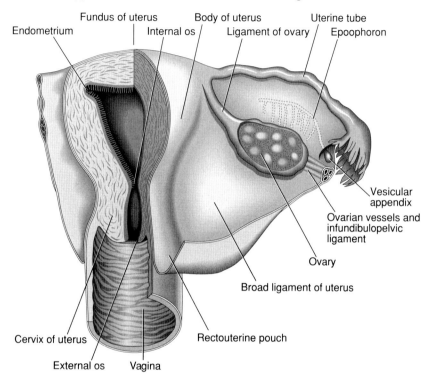

- ◆ Please refer to the textbooks listed in Further reading for more details on endometrial appearance.
  - d] Fig. 1.11b is TAS while Fig. 1.11c is TVS of an anteverted uterus and in different menstrual phase; Fig. 1.11b is TAS of an anteverted uterus while Fig. 1.11d is TAS of a retroverted uterus and in different menstrual phase.
- 12 a] Routine X-ray, hysterosalpingogram (HSG), ultrasound, laparoscopy, hysteroscopy, computed tomography (CT), magnetic resonance imaging (MRI).
  - b] • **Routine X-ray**:
    Advantages: good for demonstrating calcified fibroids; dermoids which have teeth/hair component; missing intrauterine contraceptive device (IUCD) which lies outside the uterus.
    Disadvantages: normal uterus, ovaries or tubes cannot be demonstrated; it has biological implications on an early unsuspected pregnancy.
  - • **HSG**:
    Advantages: provides reasonable diagnostic information regarding the endometrial cavity, especially that of its size, the presence of polyps and leiomyomas projecting into the endometrial cavity or distorting the cavity; good for uterine tube assessment.

A1.10c **Posterior aspect of the left broad ligament of the uterus to show the arangement of the vessels in it and the vestigial remnants of the mesonephric tubules and duct. The peritoneum of the posterior surface of the broad ligament has been removed.**

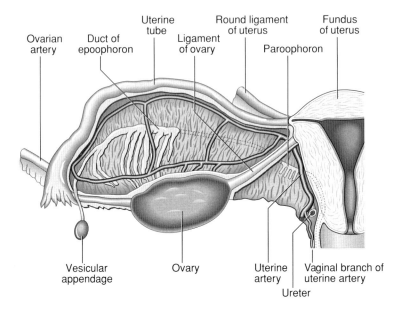

Disadvantages: uses X-radiation; has to be done at a certain time in the monthly cycle; invasive and expensive.

- ◆ HSG and hysteroscopy give almost no information regarding the myometrium per se and no diagnostic information regarding the ovaries.
- ◆ Timing of HSG in some departments is aimed at between days 10 and 20 of a new cycle when menstrual bleeding has stopped and before ovulation. The woman is equally advised to abstain from sexual intercourse from the first day of that new cycle until after the examination.

- **Ultrasound**:
  Advantages: cheaper investigation; real-time imaging is an advantage in obtaining standard planes/section for assessing and monitoring or follow up of findings/treatment; does not use X-radiation or magnetic fields; the uterus, ovaries, follicular development and ovulation and surrounding pelvic organs can be assessed at the same time; uterine tubes/endometrium can now be assessed with the use of saline or sonographic contrast media; does not require special timing, unlike HSG.
  - ◆ The recent development of sonographic contrast media and combined use of Doppler and colour flow has helped improve accuracy in the diagnosis of endometrial pathology, patency of the uterine tubes and assessment of pelvic masses.

Disadvantages: operator dependent.

- **Laparoscopy**:
  Advantages: good assessment of the pelvic organs and tubal patency with the use of the dye; may be used for diagnostic and therapeutic purposes.
  Disadvantages: high cost of procedure; surgical procedure using anaesthesia with the risk of associated complications which, although uncommon, could be serious; not cost effective for assessing and monitoring or follow up of findings/treatment.
- **Hysteroscopy**:
  Advantage: very good for endometrial evaluation.
  Disadvantages: as for laparoscopy, plus very invasive; high cost of procedure; surgical procedure using anaesthesia.
- **CT and MRI**:
  Advantage: not operator dependent.
  Disadvantages: higher cost of investigation; *CT uses X-radiation and MRI uses magnetic fields*; inflexible as the planes/sections are fixed; MRI is not available in every hospital in the UK.

13 The menstrual cycle is in two main phases – follicular and luteal – which in a regular monthly cycle are of approximately equal duration. In a 28-day cycle:

- *Follicular phase*: days 1–14. The first day of bleeding is day 1 of the cycle. Some refer to days 1–5 as the menstrual phase during which 25–65 ml of blood containing tissue fluid, mucus and epithelial cells (lining of the uterine cavity) is shed in the period. Blood flows from the uterine cavity through the vagina via the cervix. Some follicles start to develop at this time.
  Days 6–13 have been referred to by some as the preovulatory or proliferative phase. Length of this phase is subject to considerable variation in cycle length. The follicles will grow and produce more oestrogens which in turn stimulate endometrial growth and thickening. In a natural cycle one or two follicles outgrow the others, becoming the dominant follicle(s) for the month.
  Ovulation in a 28-day cycle will usually occur on day 14. At ovulation the follicle ruptures and the oocyte and follicular fluid are released. The ciliary actions of the fimbriae of the uterine tube create currents in the peritoneal serous fluid that carry the oocyte into the uterine tube. If the cycle length is short then the follicular phase will be < 14 days and vice versa.
- *Luteal or postovulatory phase*: days 15–28. This remains relatively constant at 14 days, irrespective of cycle length. Luteinizing hormone (LH) secretion stimulates the development of the corpus luteum which secretes increasing qualities of oestrogens and progesterone. Progesterone prepares the endometrium for implanatation of the blastocyst.
- Some authors prefer to describe the menstrual cycle in four phases:
  (i) menstrual phase: days 1–5
  (ii) preovulatory or proliferative or follicular phase: days 6–13
  (iii) ovulation: day 14 in a 28-day cycle
  (iv) luteal or postovulatory phase: days 15–28.

◆ Should fertilization and implantation not occur, the corpus luteum degenerates, becoming corpus albican, and the progesterone and oestrogen levels fall, thus initiating the next menstrual period.

◆ Should implantation occur, the corpus luteum continues to produce progesterone and oestrogen and this is maintained until the placenta takes over.

◆ It has been suggested that the earliest stages of follicular development appear to be controlled autonomously by the ovary and that follicular maturation and luteinization are controlled by the pituitary gland releasing the gonadotrophic hormones.

14 a] The POD is a common site for fluid collection because it is the lowest point in the pelvic cavity.

b] A small amount of fluid (10–15 mL) can be seen in the POD as a result of normal ovulation or in the periovulatory period. A larger amount of fluid can be seen in ectopic pregnancy, malignancy, ruptured ovarian cyst in children and abscesses.

15 Oocyte fertilization usually occurs in the ampulla of the uterine tube.

16 At this stage a fertilized ovum is called a zygote.

◆ Fertilization may occur up to 24 hours postovulation and the zygote reaches the uterus within 7 days.

17 A fertilized ovum descending into the uterus is called a blastocyst.

18 a] The yolk sac is seen on ultrasound between 5/40 and the end of the 1st trimester.

b] The yolk sac (YS) transfers nutrients to the embryo whilst the uteroplacental circulation is being established, i.e. between 4 and 5/40. Blood development starts in the wall of the YS and continues until haemopoiesis starts in the liver at about 8/40 gestational age (GA). By 6/40, the dorsal part of the YS is incorporated into the embryo as the primitive gut. Its endoderm forms the epithelium of the trachea, bronchi, lung and the gastrointestinal tract (GIT). Primordial germ cells appear in the YS wall by 5/40 and these later migrate to the developing sex organs.

◆ The upper limit for a normal yolk sac diameter of between 5 and 10/40 GA has been quoted as 5.6 mm.

19 The vitelline duct, also called yolk stalk or omphalomesenteric duct, connects the primitive gut to the yolk sac.

◆ The paired vitelline arteries and veins accompany the vitelline duct to provide blood supply to the yolk sac.

20 *Fig. 1.20a*

   1. Yolk sac

   2. Fetal pole

   3. Amniotic fluid

Fig. 1.20d

   10. Fetal head

   11. Limb buds

Fig. 1.20b

   4. Yolk sac

   5. Fetal pole

   6. Vitelline duct

Fig. 1.20f

   12. Cord

   13. Mid-gut herniation into the umbilical cord

Fig. 1.20c

   7. Cord

   8. Yolk sac

   9. Vitelline duct

Fig. 1.20g
14. Prosencephalon (forebrain)
15. Mesencephalon (midbrain)
16. Rhombencephalon (hindbrain)

Fig. 1.20h
17. Yolk sac
18. Amnion

Fig. 1.20i
a. Foot
b. Cord
c. Cord
d. Amnion
e. Fetal head
f. Yolk sac
g. Uterine wall

Fig. 1.20j
19. Knee
20. Foot
21. Bottom/bum
22. Intestine
23. Spine
24. Diaphragm
25. Heart
26. Mandible
27. Choroid plexus

Fig. 1.20k
28. Eye socket
29. Thumb
30. Index finger
31. Middle finger
32. Ring finger
33. Little finger
34. Radius
35. Ulna

b] The fetus is 8–9/40. This is because the limb buds are just becoming visible.

c] Measurement is of crown–rump length (CRL).

21 • *Embryonic period*: from fertilization to 8 weeks after fertilization. (Changes appearing at this period are dramatic/rapid and the embryo is more vulnerable to the teratogenic effects of drugs, viruses and radiation.)

• *Fetal period*: begins at 9 weeks after fertilization, i.e. 11 weeks after the last menstrual period (LMP) until birth. (During the fetal period there is rapid body growth and differentiation of tissues and organ systems. Whilst the fetus is less vulnerable to the effects of teratogenic drugs, viruses and radiation, these agents may interfere with fetal growth and normal functional development, especially the brain and eyes.)

22 a] Chromosomes are thread-like bodies seen in all living cells; they carry genetic material (e.g. genes and other DNA).

b] The genes carry hereditary information responsible for cell function and physical characteristics.

c] At fertilization the ovum and sperm contribute 23 chromosomes each. The individual thus receives 23 pairs of chromosomes from both parents. These may be made up from normal and/or abnormal genes.

d] Genetic abnormality may be spontaneous (e.g. a chance error or division or replication) or induced by exposure to environmental mutagenic agents such as chemicals, radiation and temperature.

♦ Radiation, drugs, chemicals and viruses can induce chromosome breaks; the resulting abnormality of the chromosome is dependent on what happens to the broken pieces.

♦ It has been suggested that exposing the embryo during development to large doses of X-radiation or radium in the 1st trimester may cause microcephaly, skeletal malformation and mental retardation.

b] *Fig. 1.61a*: normal 4-chamber (4C) view obtained with the ultrasound beam perpendicular to the interventricular septum.

Fig. 1.61b: normal 4C view.

Fig. 1.61c: sagittal view showing the descending aorta.

62 a] TORCH stands for a group of infections which may affect the fetus, i.e. *T*oxoplasmosis, *R*ubella (German measles), *C*ytomegalovirus and *H*erpes.

b] Ultrasound-recognizable effects of TORCH in utero:
— toxoplasmosis may cause intrauterine death (IUD), microcephaly, hydrocephalus, intracranial calcification
— rubella can cause IUGR, congenital heart disease (fetal infection with rubella is uncommon if at the time of maternal infection the fetus is > 20/40 GA)
— cytomegalovirus can cause microcephaly, intracranial calcification, hepatoslenomegaly, IUGR.

63 a] The rare VATER syndrome is a group of associated abnormalities of unknown origin, neither chromosomally related nor familial:

V – vascular; dextrocardia, ventricular septal defect

A – anorectal atresia

T – tracheo-oesophageal fistula

E – oesophageal atresia

R – renal abnormalities, radial absence.

b] In suspected VATER syndrome the fetal bowel, arms and heart should be checked.

64 *Fig. 1.64a*　　　　*Fig. 1.64b*　　　　　*Fig. 1.64c*

Fig. 1.64a	*Fig. 1.64b*	*Fig. 1.64c*
1. Penis	4. Fetal thigh	6. Urinary bladder
2. Testis	5. Labial folds	7. Penis
3. Scrotum		8. Fetal thigh

65 a] *Fig. 1.65a*　　　　　*Fig. 1.65b*

Fig. 1.65a	*Fig. 1.65b*
1. Umbilical vein	3. Umbilical artery
2. Umbilical artery	4. Umbilical vein

b] Fig. 1.65a shows a sagittal/longitudinal section of a three-vessel umbilical cord.

Fig. 1.65b shows a TS of a three-vessel umbilical cord (see Answer 46 above).

c] i] Transvaginal scan was used to obtain this image.

ii] In Fig. 1.65c, a = maternal urinary bladder, b = amniotic fluid, c = fetal head and d = cervical canal.

iii] Measurement + to + is of cervical length.

Physics and instrumentation

ANSWERS

1 a] Humans perceive sound frequencies between 20 Hz and 20 kHz. Ultrasound is sound which has a frequency above this and which is therefore beyond normal human hearing. In medical imaging the sound frequencies used are in the range of 1–10 MHz (3.5–7.5 MHz is usual in obstetrics and gynaecology). 1 MHz = 1 000 000 Hz.

   b] When the piezoelectric crystal(s) is activated electronically, pulses of sound at very high frequencies (ultrasound) are produced.

   c] Coupling gel is used to eliminate air, i.e. decreasing the acoustic impedance and thus promoting good transmission of ultrasound from the transducer to soft tissue and vice versa. Gels are mostly water soluble or olive oil.

   d] It is important to use only the gel suitable for a transducer as indicated by the manufacturer in order to avoid transducer damage.

   ◆ Answers given to patients should be tailored to their perceived level of understanding.

2 a] Noise is a disorderly transmission of mechanical vibrations through a medium, while sound is the orderly transmission of same.

   b] • Amplitude of a waveform (A) is the height of the apex of the oscillation above the baseline.
   • Wavelength (λ) is the distance between two consecutive, equivalent points on a waveform.
   • Frequency measured in hertz (Hz) is the number of vibrations/waves that occur in 1 second.

3 Piezoelectric effect is a phenomenon seen when electrical current is applied to each side of a piece of quartz coated with silver. The quartz expands or contracts from its original thickness, depending on the polarity of the current applied.

4 Ultrasound frequency is determined by the thickness of the piezoelectric element.

5 Resonant frequency is the frequency at which a piezoelectric element vibrates when an alternating current is applied to it. This stable frequency is governed/determined by the thickness of the element.

6 When alternating current is applied to each surface of the piezoelectric material, ultrasound is produced and vibrates at a stable frequency; when the piezoelectric material is physically compressed by externally applied ultrasound it produces a current.

7 Speed of sound in soft tissues varies between 1500 and 1600 metres per second (m/s). Velocity on current ultrasound equipment is standardized at 1540 m/s.

8 In TA the beam direction is from anterior to posterior, whereas in TVS it is from caudal to cephalic.

9 Intensity of ultrasound is decreased by scatter, absorption and reflection (SAR).

10 • Scatter: when the beam encounters an interface that is irregular or smaller than the ultrasound beam, it is scattered in all directions.

    • Tissue absorption: increases with increasing frequency of the ultrasound beam. This is important when scanning small parts (e.g. thyroid, testis, breast) where a high frequency probe is used; probe frequency should match the type of investigation and patient size.

    • Reflection: occurs when the ultrasound beam passes from a tissue of one acoustic impedance to a tissue of a different impedance. It requires a smooth surface which is larger than the wavelength of the beam. Only reflected ultrasound is used for medical imaging.

    ♦ The contour of the tissue or organ being scanned is determined by reflection, whereas the inner echo pattern is primarily determined by scatter.

11 All SAR elements contribute to decreasing the intensity of the ultrasound beam.

12 Refraction is the bending of the ultrasound beam when it crosses the interface of tissues of different acoustic impedance at an oblique angle.

13 The beam should be perpendicular to the interface because most of the reflected beam comes back to the transducer yielding a strong signal.

14 a] Focal length is the distance from the transducer face to the focal zone.

    b] The Fresnel zone, or near field, is the area close to the transducer where the ultrasound beam is uneven; the Fraunhofer zone, or far field, is the area where the transmitted ultrasound beam begins to diverge.

    c] The points in Fig. A2.14 comprise:

a. Cable	c. Crystal	e. Focal length	g. Focal zone.
b. Transducer	d. Focal point	f. Beam diverging	

15 a] Beam/transducer focusing is a method by which the width of the ultrasound beam may be regulated and the region of maximum density adjusted.

    b] Ultrasound beam focusing is achieved by using a transducer with a concave face (internal focusing) or by placing an acoustic lens in front of the piezoelectric crystal (external focusing).

    ♦ Focusing can also be achieved using the quarter wavelength theory.

16 In electronic focusing changing the timing of probe element firing produces a change in focal distance or beam direction.

17 Resolution is the ability to separate two small objects placed close together. There are two types of resolution: axial and lateral. Factors such as frequency, pulse length, transducer geometry and focusing affect resolution.

18 • *Axial resolution* is the ability to distinguish between structures in line with the ultrasound beam. Determined by dampening (ringdown) and wavelength, axial resolution is approximately 1 mm at 3.5 MHz.

- *Lateral resolution* is the ability to separate two objects in a plane perpendicular to the beam. The narrower the beam, the better the lateral resolution. It is best at a distance equal to the focal length.

19 • **Linear electronic or linear array**: the transducer face is 5–12 cm, but most often 8 cm, composed of 60–130 thin, regular crystals. To produce a focused beam, 7–8 crystals are used as a group. Varying the time at which individual crystals are fired, with the more central crystals delayed relative to the outer ones, the ultrasound beam from this group focuses to form a narrow beam.
  Electronic focusing occurs in longitudinal direction of the transducer while mechanical focusing occurs in the direction of the short axis by using an acoustic lens.
  Advantages: good for obstetric work, demonstrating long linear structures (e.g. aorta) or superficial structures (e.g. pleural cavity).
  Disadvantages: relatively small visual field compared to contact scanner with consequent difficulty in identifying the orientation.

- **Contact compound**: the transducer head is moved manually to image a cross-section of the patient. The position and direction of the transducer are calculated by the angles of the three joints of the arm to which the transducer is attached.
  Advantage: areas partially obscured by the ribs and gas are effectively demonstrated as well as organ relationships.
  Disadvantages: suffers from motion artefact; skill is required to obtain good smooth images; only static images can be obtained and the equipment is expensive.

- **Phased array**: same principle as linear electronic.
  Advantages: the beam can be electronically steered; the transducer is smaller; suitable for intercostal examination of liver and indispensable for pelvis.
  Disadvantages: more expensive than the linear array because of more complicated electrical circuitry to produce accurate timing; because each piezoelectric crystal is approximately half the size of those in the linear array, they are more difficult to manufacture.

- **Convex and electronic (curved linear)**: similar to linear but with convex surface. Ultrasound beam always perpendicular to the surface of the transducer head. Superficial structures better imaged than with electronic sector scanner due to longer transducer face. Angle of beam spread usually 60° but close to 100° in microconvex type.
  Advantage: they have good resolution.

- **Mechanical sector**: fan-shaped image produced from three or four transducers mounted on a wheel that is rotated, a single transducer which rocks back and forth within the transducer head, or a single stationary transducer where the beam is moved by an oscillating mirror which reflects the sound (less expensive).
  Advantages: good for intercostal scanning and aortic aneurysm demonstration.
  Disadvantages: fixed focal zone and vibration felt by the operator.

Gynaecology

ANSWERS

1 Much time is spent in patient contact. Good communication with the patient helps to:
 — allay patient anxiety and fears
 — reassure the patient
 — elicit pertinent information from the patient which may not be written on the request card
 — promote rapport with the patient prior to and during the examination.
 ◆ It is not uncommon to have a time lapse between the date a routine gynaecology scan is requested and the examination is actually performed. There is therefore a need to re-clarify the clinical history and note any changes that might have occurred in the interim.
 ◆ Thorough knowledge of pelvic pathology, being able to listen to and interpret a patient's symptoms and obtain the relevant past clinical history are essential.

2 Determining the source of tenderness helps to relate it with the organ that lies directly beneath the localized area of tenderness. This may indicate, for example, the presence of an ongoing infection.

3

Question	Reason for enquiry
a. When was your last menstrual period?	Helps in clarifying the ultrasound appearances and therefore the decision (e.g. type of cystic area in the ovary)
b. Was the bleeding normal in duration and amount?	An abnormally light bleed could be associated with threatened abortion, an ectopic or a normal pregnancy. A heavier than normal bleed may be associated with an incomplete abortion or pelvic inflammatory disease (PID)
c. Were there any blood clots?	Blood clots could be seen in abortion or in patients with fibroids, with or without any associated pain
d. Would you describe your menstrual period as regular or irregular; how many days are there between one period and another period?	Helps in clarifying the ultrasound appearances and therefore the possible differential diagnosis
e. What contraceptive method, if any, do you use?	Patients who conceive whilst wearing an intrauterine contraceptive device (IUCD) or while taking the progesterone-only pill are particularly at risk of an ectopic pregnancy
f. Have you been on any sort of fertility treatment?	There is an increased risk of heterotopic pregnancy associated with ovulation induction or assisted reproduction techniques
g. Have you had any pelvic surgery before?	Patients with previous tubal surgery are prone to ectopic pregnancy, and in patients with previous oophorectomy there is no need to spend time looking for an already removed ovary(ies)

Questions asked will depend on the age of the patient and the reason for the scan, for example questions e and f are irrelevant for a postmenopausal woman.

4 TVS is target oriented whereas TA scan is governed by the ultrasound planes. For TA scan the ultrasound waves are transmitted from the abdomen to the back (ventral to dorsal) whereas in TVS, transmission is from the feet to the head (caudal to cephalic).

5 Ultrasound is useful in the management of pelvic mass when:
   — clinical examination is impossible due to acute pain or obesity
   — it is unclear whether the mass is ovarian or uterine
   — it is uncertain whether the mass is solid or cystic
   — accurate size measurement is necessary
   — assessing the effect of the pelvic mass on the other pelvic structures and on the kidneys and liver
   — undertaking follow-up assessment of the mass.

6 Clinical indications for TVS include:
   — evaluation of the uterine cavity/fallopian tube assessment ultrasound using normal saline or saline-based antibiotic preparations or other solutions of low echogenicity or echogenic contrast media-based solution (e.g. HyCoSy)
   — evaluation of gynaecological conditions
   — evaluation of the ovaries for ovarian disease and in those women with a high risk for ovarian cancer
   — infertility/hormone therapy
   — 1st trimester fetal evaluation
   — 1st trimester pregnancy complications assessment
   — 3rd trimester lower uterine segment evaluation
   — exclusion of ectopic pregnancy
   — investigation for endometrial pathology in postmenopausal women
   — evaluation of translabial and vaginal urinary tract.

7 Contraindications to TVS include:
   — no previous history of sexual activity
   — heavy vaginal bleeding, especially in early pregnancy
   — suspicion of cervical incompetence, especially in patients presenting in early pregnancy
   — patients under 18 years of age
   — certain ethnic or religious groups
   — evidence of stress or anxiety towards this type of examination
   — history of repeated early miscarriage.

8 TVS can provide additional information when there is need to differentiate between:
   — cystic or solid structure
   — simple or complex structure
   — ovarian or uterine structure
   — ovarian or tubal entity
   — free fluid or fluid in the bowels
   — fibroid or retroverted uterus.

22

Ovarian cyst	Hydrosalpinx
Always round sonographically	Tubular, 'sausage shaped' or coily
No space between the ovary and cyst except in paraovarian cyst which is separable from the ovary	Occasionally possible to have a space between the ovary and the hydrosalpinx
Functional cyst usually resolves later (may be up to 10 weeks)	Always persistent
Convex wall adjacent to the ovary	Convex wall away from the ovary and concave wall adjacent to the ovary
Septum (where seen) is single walled	Double-wall sign
Nodularity seen in malignancies	Thickened mucosal folds do not extend from wall to wall

Scanning the structure from all sides and observing its shape and relationship with the ovary and the other pelvic structures may be helpful in distinguishing between the two conditions.
Modified with permission from Dodson M G 1995 Transvaginal ultrasound, 2nd edn. Churchill Livingstone, New York.

23 Conditions associated with increased fluid in the pouch of Douglas

Non-gynaecological conditions	Gynaecological conditions
Appendicitis	Gynaecological pathology
Abdominal infections	PID
Intra-abdominal bleeding post-trauma (e.g. ruptured spleen)	OHSS
Non-gynaecological cancer (e.g. intra-abdominal cancer)	Ruptured ectopic pregnancy

Some free fluid may be seen normally in the POD premenstruation and around the mid-cycle due to released fluid from the follicle, especially in non-oral contraceptive users.

24 With fresh blood clots, there will usually be irregular hypoechoic masses with increased fluid in the POD. With old blood, the mass will be irregular but hyperechoic in structure and appearance.
  ◆ Sonographic appearance of blood is determined by the time that has lapsed between the bleeding and when the scan is performed.
25 The ovaries are not normally glued to the uterus, so it is possible during transvaginal scan (TVS) to use the probe gently to push them away from the uterus in normal cases. However, in patients with pelvic adhesions, there will be an en bloc motion of contiguous viscera rather than independent motion of the individual organs, affecting the motility of the ovaries in relationship with the uterus.
26 Endometriosis and chronic pelvic inflammatory disease are associated with bilateral adnexal masses.
27 Using real-time ultrasound, peristalsis will be noted in cases of fluid- or stool-filled bowel. Water enema can be used to demonstrate fluid entering the rectosigmoid. Rescanning the patient at short-term follow up will demonstrate a change in the configuration of bowel loops which are not adherent.

28 With pelvic ascites, the uterus will be clearly outlined as it will fill the anterior and posterior POD. The superior uterine border will be irregular due to gut indentations, whereas the superior border of the urinary bladder will be smooth. The urinary bladder will decrease in size after the patient has voided but the appearance of pelvic ascites is not affected by voiding.

29 A woman may have her uterus removed but ovaries retained because of:
— menorrhagia (e.g. secondary to bleeding from fibroids with no disease of the ovaries)
— endometriosis covering the outside of the uterus and cardinal ligaments
— menstrual problems without involvement of the ovaries in which medical and less invasive surgical intervention has failed to improve the situation.
♦ The fact that a woman (especially one of childbearing age) has had a hysterectomy does not necessarily mean she does not have her ovaries still in place.

30 Pelvic examination may be difficult to perform due to the patient's discomfort in PID.

31 Ultrasound can:
— demonstrate the presence of disease, the extent of an inflammatory process, and the response to therapy
— be used to determine the best route for drainage (abscess, cyst, etc.)
— be used to confirm or disprove postoperative collections following surgery.

32 Using the transvaginal (TV) route, pyosalpinx is seen as a smooth-walled curving tubular structure with a club shape. The fluid collection is echogenic due to low level echoes.

33 Pyosalpinx appearance is defined in Answer 32 above. In hydrosalpinx the fallopian tube is fluid-filled and tortuous, extending from the cornua.

34 A pelvic abscess appears on ultrasound as a cystic mass with a variable amount of internal debris and with an irregular wall. The mass may be poorly circumscribed due to contiguous inflammation and may displace adjacent structures.
♦ Some abscesses may contain highly echogenic centres which may cause acoustic shadowing.

35 In a pelvic scan of the urinary bladder the presence or absence of the following should be noted:
— bladder wall
— calculi
— diverticulum
— indentation/displacement by any pelvic mass or cyst
— bladder wall thickening
— any other abnormal finding.

36 Calcification of the arcuate artery usually involves multiple vessels at about the same level in the myometrium. This tends to form a linear configuration on a longitudinal image of an anteroposterior (AP) pelvis or a circular configuration in the transverse section (TS).

- With fibroma the calcification is seen as randomly distributed in the fibroid or at the periphery and outlining the fibroid.

37 It has been suggested that there is an association between arcuate artery calcification and atherosclerotic disease and diabetes or hypertension. Further clinical investigation for such underlying problems is warranted.

38 A haematoma or loss of the uterine wall integrity is suggestive of uterine rupture. There may also be an echopoor area with echogenic material (fetal material) in the uterovesical space.

39 Gynaecological ultrasound can be of use:
— in patients with a large uterus or those with a large amount of tissue that must be removed, especially where there is a thin uterine wall
— in guiding endometrial biopsies in patients with stenotic endocervical canals
— for dilation and curettage or suction curettage to help to determine the location of the curette or suction cannula and to locate tissue in the uterine cavity. This will help to prevent perforation while ensuring that the uterine cavity has been evaluated or evacuated adequately.

40 Patients with Turner's syndrome have a small uterus, which is prepubertal in shape; they also have small ovaries (< 1 cm^3).

41 Ovarian malignancy may be suggested by:
— a mass or masses which may be of any nature from pure cystic to pure solid, with multiloculations, thick septa (especially if incomplete), with or without nodules, the presence of papillary projections, ill-defined margins, and thick walls; such mass(es) are also persistent
— ascites
— invasion of the uterus by the ovarian mass.
- Ideally, simple follicular cysts tend to disappear when scanned in another menstrual phase (e.g. in 6 weeks) but may be seen for up to 10 weeks after the previous scan. Ovarian malignancy does not disappear.
- Blood flow is seen in most ovarian malignancies, with high velocity, low impedance blood flow, demonstrating forward flow throughout the cardiac cycle and decreased pulsatility index (PI) and resistance index (RI). Although no definite value has been fixed, it has been suggested that a PI of 1.0 and a RI of ≤ 0.4 may give a high predictive value and low false negative value.
- In most malignancies, there will be blood flow seen within the centre of the lesion.
- Blood flow is seen in the periphery of most benign lesions; some lesions, however, show flow within the centre of the lesion.

42 Dermoid could present on ultrasound as:
— a cyst with a fat–fluid level
— an echogenic mass within a cystic lesion
— echogenic particles within a low echogenic fluid background.

43 In pelvic mass the following should be documented:
— number and size of mass(es)
— nature of the mass, i.e. overall echogenicity

— margins – regular or irregular, thin or thick walled
— cystic or solid component
— reflective shadowing
— position of the mass in relation to other pelvic organs, i.e. urinary bladder, uterus and ovaries
— ultrasonic appearance of the uterus and ovaries (if seen)
— if the mass is putting pressure on or invading the pelvic organs
— pelvic or abdominal ascites
— Kidney size and any sign of hydronephrosis or hydroureters
— liver state and the presence of metastases or enlarged lymph nodes (depending on departmental protocol).

44 A simple ovarian cyst may appear as an echolucent mass, with a thin, well-defined posterior wall, with posterior wall enhancement.
   ♦ Ideally, simple follicular cysts tend to disappear when scanned in another menstrual phase (e.g. 6 weeks later) but may be seen for up to 10 weeks.

45 On ultrasound an endometrioma may appear as:
   — a complex mass with debris or internal septation or internal echoes
   — a purely cystic mass
   — a solid mass.
   ♦ Clinically most patients with endometrioma may present with dysmenorrhoea, pre- and postmenstrual pains, deep dyspareunia, menorrhagia, spotting and intramenstrual bleeding (IMB).
   ♦ Endometriosis occurs during the reproductive years.

46 Bicornuate uterus is suggested by the presence of:
   — double endometrial cavity which is best seen on TS
   — interrupted endometrial echoes in the TS
   — uterine dimensions of more than 8 cm on the TS.

47 • During the menstrual phase (days 1–5) the endometrium appears as a thin echogenic line measuring 2–3 mm in thickness.
   • During the proliferative phase (days 6–13) the endometrium begins to thicken, becoming slightly hyperechoic and measuring 4–6 mm in thickness.
   • Just prior to and after ovulation an inner hyperechoic line is seen in the endometrium; this is referred to as the 'triple stripe' and occasionally a small amount of fluid may be seen.
   • During the secretory or luteal phase the endometrium is thick and echogenic, measuring 8–12 mm in thickness (see also Answer 13 in Chapter 1).

48 A normal menopausal endometrium is thin and smooth, measuring 1–3 mm in thickness.
   ♦ It is not uncommon to find an absent endometrial echo in postmenopausal women who are not on hormone replacement therapy (HRT) 15–20 years after the menopause.

49 In endometrial assessment an ultrasound scan is useful in evaluating:
   — underlying pelvic pathology
   — polyp
   — hyperplasia

   — endometrial cancer

   — the endometrium by distension with fluid.

It is also useful in assessing endometrial response during fertility treatment.

50 Endometrial motion may correlate with the menstrual cycle physiology and/or sexual function. The uterus in a sexually mature individual is never motionless. Endometrial movement is most pronounced 2–3 days after sexual intercourse, with retrograde movement from the cervix towards the fundus; this is also seen in early pregnancy. Antegrade movement, i.e. from the fundus towards the cervix, is seen during menstruation and has been seen in patients with inevitable abortion.

Movement increases throughout the follicular phase and into the periovulatory period and then decreases until menstruation. Most movement is seen in in vitro fertilization (IVF) patients and least movement in patients with a natural cycle.

51 a] Abnormal uterine bleeding is menstrual bleeding which is not normal in nature, for example postmenopausal bleed, bleeding between periods with no prior warning, too frequent bleeding (e.g. two periods in a month), diminished blood flow or excessive blood flow with clots during menstruation.

   b] Abnormal uterine bleeding may be due to adenomyosis, fibroid tumours, systemic disease, disordered hormonal regulation or endometrial pathology.

   c] Ultrasound can be used to assess the uterus, ovaries and pelvis to find an identifiable anatomical cause for the abnormal uterine bleeding.

52 Patients on COC have a thickened single line, 3–5 mm thick, hyperechoic endometrium, better described as a thick single line endometrium or a very thin luteal phase endometrium. This is not the same as the single line, 1–3 mm, single line thin endometrium seen at the time of menstruation. This thickening in patients on COC reflects the endometrial response to simultaneous stimulation with both oestrogen and progesterone.

♦ Patients on COC may sometimes have breakthrough bleeding.

♦ The same appearance may be seen in postmenopausal women on oestrogen replacement therapy when combined with progesterone.

53 Causes of a hyperechoic endometrium include:

   — endometrial cancer

   — adenomatous hyperplasia

   — polyps or fibroids projecting into the endometrium

   — early pregnancy before the gestational sac (GS) is visible

   — ectopic pregnancy

   — incomplete abortion

   — RPOC

   — trophoblastic disease.

♦ The presenting clinical history of the patient will help in eliminating the least likely cause in each case.

54 Such endometrial findings can be seen in patients with PCOD, chronic anovulation with chronic low level oestrogen stimulation and/or long-term menometrorrhagia or hyperplasia.

55 In triple line endometrium the sonographer should also check the ovaries because follicles could develop and ovulation is not uncommon. Follicle, corpus luteal cyst or oestrogen-producing cyst or tumour needs to be excluded.

56 A mixed echo endometrium will demonstrate both hypo- and hyperechoic appearances. This may be associated with submucosal fibroids or endometrial polyps, incomplete abortion or where there is a mixture of blood and tissue in the endometrial cavity.

57 Absent endometrium is typically seen in postmenopausal women and sometimes in women on birth control pills.

58 The typical appearance of an anechoic endometrium is of a fluid-filled structure with a thin hyperechoic rim. The fluid could be blood or fluid during a normal menstruation, secondary to cervical stenosis, or cancer of the cervix, especially in postmenopausal women who ought not to be having a period.

59 Luteal phase endometrium may be seen:
— where a corpus luteal cyst (CLC) is present but does not produce adequate progesterone to support the endometrium
— in early pregnancy or in pregnancy complications (including ectopic pregnancy)
— in polyps
— in fibroids
— in RPOC.

60 Routine scan prior to insertion of an IUCD is recommended in patients at risk of malplacement (e.g. obese or postpartum women) and in women with a retroflexed or retroverted uterus who are at risk of perforation.

61 Clinical indications for an ultrasound scan after insertion of an IUCD include:
— lost string or lost IUCD
— cramping pain
— abnormal bleeding
— pregnancy with IUCD in situ
— possible perforation
— possible misplaced IUCD
— positive pregnancy test result with known IUCD in situ.
♦ It has been suggested that IUCD users are at greater risk of PID than non-users and sometimes a 'silent' tubo-ovarian abscess may be seen.
♦ Ovulation and CLC formation are not suppressed with IUCD use, thus users have the same risk of developing simple ovarian cysts.

62 In scanning for IUCD localization, the following should be recorded:
— the presence or absence of the IUCD within the uterus
— the position of the IUCD within the uterus (ideally it should be situated in the fundal area of the cavity with the entire device distal to the internal cervical os)
— outcome of the study of both adnexal areas, ruling out or confirming the presence of a coexisting extrauterine pregnancy.

63 In pregnancy with an IUCD in situ, it is essential to ascertain the relationship of the device to the gestational sac (i.e. superior or inferior) and to obtain a trimester scan report of the embryo/fetus in line with departmental protocol.

64 A properly placed IUCD will remove the possibility of the IUCD's expulsion, severe cramping and bleeding. In addition, contraceptive effectiveness will be optimal.

65 When ultrasound fails to detect a missing IUCD, a plain abdominal X-ray may be used. If the X-ray confirms the IUCD in the pelvis a hysterosalpingogram (HSG) can be performed to confirm its specific location.
   ♦ All the above techniques have biological implications on an early unsuspected pregnancy.

66 An embedded IUCD is suspected when:
   — there is an eccentrically placed IUCD in the uterus
   — the central uterine cavity echo which represents the endometrium is not seen surrounding the IUCD.
   ♦ Fibroids, bicornuate uterus and other congenital uterine abnormalities may complicate localization of the IUCD.

67 a] Partial perforation by an IUCD is indicated by an incomplete echo pattern of the IUCD.
   b] Complete perforation by an IUCD is indicated by non-visualization of the IUCD in the uterus despite radiographic evidence of the device in the pelvis.
   ♦ Partial perforation occurs when part of the IUCD is still within the myometrium.

68 To confirm a non-Mirena IUCD in the uterus, turn down the postprocessing or the overall gain setting on the ultrasound equipment and the device will still be visible.

69 Retained bone fragments from an incomplete abortion can mimic an IUCD in the uterus.

70 a] An IUCD in a retroverted or retroflexed uterus may not be recognized on ultrasound because the ultrasound beam may not be in the optimum axis in relation to the IUCD for proper visualization, thus the typical acoustical shadowing may not be demonstrated.
   b] Recognition of an IUCD in a retroverted or retroflexed uterus may be assisted by:
   — having the patient fill her bladder adequately (for transabdominal (TA) approach)
   — manual manipulation of the uterus during the scan by the gynaecologist.

71 a] On a transverse section (TS) of the uterus, the arm of the Copper 7 coil joins the shaft at one end; the arm of the Copper T coil joins the shaft at the middle.
   b] On the longitudinal section of the uterus, the Mirena coil displays two bright echoes near the cervical os and a third echo at the fundus. In the transverse view angled towards the fundus, parallel echogenic lines are seen.
   c] The Mirena coil is difficult to identify on ultrasound because it contains barium sulphate instead of copper as in other IUCDs. It is therefore less opaque on ultrasound but can be seen on X-ray images as barium sulphate is opaque.

d] If TAS fails to demonstrate a missing Mirena coil, TVS should be tried.

◆ It is advisable to ask the woman which type of coil is being sought prior to the start of the examination.

◆ IUCDs containing copper may give a 'comet tail' artefact.

◆ The Mirena intrauterine system may be more difficult to identify than the other types of IUCD as it is less echogenic.

◆ The Mirena coil (in use since 1995) contains progestogen (levonorgestrel) which is released at a rate of 20 μg/24 hours. It contains barium sulphate but no metal.

72 Risks with the use of an IUCD include:

— PID

— ectopic/heterotopic pregnancy

— spontaneous abortion

— actinomycosis infection of the uterus with unreplaced, long-term use of an IUCD.

73 a] A leiomyoma is a benign smooth-muscle tumour of the uterus, sometimes called a fibroid. The fibrous tissue content is variable. Apart from pregnancy, it is the commonest cause of uterine enlargement, common in women over 35 years old, and more common in the African-Caribbean race. It is hormone dependent, associated with high oestrogen levels, and may grow bigger during pregnancy and with the use of HRT and tamoxifen therapy. Leiomyomas tend to shrink postmenopausally, with the use of oral contraceptive pills and with the use of gonadotrophin releasing hormone antagonists which may be prescribed prior to myomectomy or hysterectomy.

b] • Leiomyomas may be in the anterior or posterior fundal wall of the uterus or outside the uterus, i.e. pedunculated.

• Submucosal leiomyomas lie adjacent to the uterine cavity. Estimated to be about 5% of all leiomyomas, they are the most symptomatic, presenting with abnormal per vaginal (PV) bleeding, dysmenorrhoea and menorrhagia. A cause for an increase in endometrium area, they may prevent pregnancy implantation or cause recurrent miscarriages (1st or 2nd trimester abortion), premature labour or abnormal presentation. They may hinder endometrial nutrition which may result in poor placentation leading to intrauterine growth retardation (IUGR).

• Subserosal leiomyomas lie on the outer uterine surface.

• Intramural leiomyomas lie in the intermediate or intramyometrial position.

• Pedunculated leiomyomas arise from the outside wall of the uterus. They may twist and become painful.

◆ Leiomyomas that lie in the cervical area may obstruct labour.

◆ A small leiomyoma within the endometrium may cast acoustic shadows, thus differentiating it from an endometrial polyp which is typically hyperechoic.

◆ The differentials of each leiomyoma will depend on its position.

c] Fig. 3.73c – fibroid location:

a – pedunculated

b – fundal*

       c – posterior*

       d – submucosal

       e – anterior**

       f – anterior cervical

       g – posterior cervical.

       * intramural leiomyoma; ** subserosal leiomyoma.

74 A known leiomyoma is scanned in order to:

— confirm that a clinically detected mass is not an ovarian neoplasm

— detect cervical leiomyomas in pregnancy

— monitor the size of a leiomyoma, especially after menopause

— aid in the differential diagnosis of abdominal pain.

75 Leiomyoma is suggested by the presence of a diffused enlarged uterus, homogenous except where there is fibroid degeneration, in which case there may be cystic or echogenic areas, uterine outline irregularity, calcifications with shadowing, an altered echo texture, localized uterine enlargement and indefinite uterus; the urinary bladder wall may be indented by anterior wall leiomyoma(s).

- A large leiomyoma may compress the ureter(s) or urinary bladder and thus cause unilateral or bilateral hydronephrosis.
- Increase in size of a leiomyoma in the absence of pregnancy, the use of HRT or tamoxifen therapy is suggestive of malignancy.
- Malignant changes in a leiomyoma are very rare.
- High velocity blood flow may be seen, especially within large leiomyomas, but the flow pattern and impedance values obtained vary considerably.
- TAS and TVS when used together can help in confirming and assessing leiomyomas and in ruling out bicornuate or retroverted uterus.
- Calcification is noted in about 25% of leiomyomas on ultrasound.

76 With leiomyomas, uterine wall outline distortion is permanent whereas with Braxton Hicks contractions the distortion or bunching up will disappear after approximately 30 minutes.

77 Leiomyomas may grow rapidly and outstrip their blood supply, leading to central degeneration. In pregnancy, bleeding into the centre of the leiomyoma is called *red degeneration*, which can be acutely painful. The woman will be tender over the exact site of the leiomyoma. Current leiomyoma measurement will be larger than the previous measurement.

Bleeding into the centre of a leiomyoma in a non-pregnant woman is called *hyaline degeneration* and is mostly painless. Ultrasonically this appears as an echo-free area within the leiomyoma.

- Torsion of a pedunculated leiomyoma, or haemorrhage within it, may cause acute pain.

78 After menopause leiomyomas usually decrease in size due to reduction in hormone levels. A size increase may suggest malignancy.

79 Where the leiomyoma extends out of the pelvis, a TA scan will provide more information than a TVS. The kidneys could also be assessed with a TA scan to confirm or exclude hydronephrosis.

80 Differential diagnosis of leiomyomas (fibroids) and adenomyosis

Leiomyomas	Adenomyosis
Nodular heterogeneous structures with well-defined borders	Heterogeneous circumscribed area of the myometrium with indistinct margins Irregular cystic spaces 5–7 mm in size, i.e. honeycomb or polycystic myometrium, thought to consist of blood-containing cavities
Contour irregularity	Disruption of homogeneous echo pattern
Diffuse uterine enlargement	Diffuse uterine enlargement
Indefinite uterus	Thickened posterior wall of uterus
Altered echo texture	Eccentric endometrial cavity
Calcification with shadowing	Hyperechoic density with acoustic shadows

◆ Adenomyosis can present in two forms: diffuse or focal. Diffuse adenomyosis results in involvement of the entire myometrium and thus symmetrical uterine enlargement. In focal adenomyosis, the ectopic endometrium is surrounded by smooth hypertrophied muscle, thus appearing as a circumscribed nodule which may look like a leiomyoma.

81 a] Postmenopausal bleeding is frequently associated with pelvic pathology. Abnormalities are reported in 20–33% of patients, with 5–10% having endometrial cancer. In the UK, postmenopausal bleeding is quoted as accounting for up to 5% of gynaecology outpatients.

b] Causes of postmenopausal bleeding include polyps, hyperplasia and intracavity fluid.
  ◆ The thickness of the intracavity fluid must be distinguished from true endometrial thickening. This is done by measuring the fluid separately. The ultrasound appearance of the fluid should be described (e.g. pyometra).

82 Postmenopausal ovaries can be difficult to locate because of their small size (average 1.5 cm³) and lack of anechoic follicles.

83 Ovarian problems in a postmenopausal patient may include:
  — ovarian volume of more than 10 ml (some authors quote 5 cm³)
  — discrepancy in the sizes of the ovaries (ideally the ovaries should be approximately the same size, the volume of one being no more than twice that of the other)
  — any cystic structure in the ovary irrespective of the woman being on HRT, especially after 5 years of becoming menopausal.
  ◆ Follicles that develop within the first 5 years after becoming menopausal tend to disappear, just as they would in a normal cycle when there is no pathology.

84 a] A mucocele is a mucus-filled appendix. It usually appears as an echogenic mass, most often ovoid in shape.
  b] In mucocele/ovarian dermoid differentiation, a careful scan will demonstrate a normal right ovary when it is a mucocele.

85 A woman of child-bearing age with a history of previous hysterectomy would/could be referred for a pelvic scan:
  — to rule out/confirm pelvic collections/abscess following surgery

— to find cause of pelvic pains

— to find out cause of pelvic bleed if the cervix was left behind at surgery

— to assess the ovaries if they were left behind

— to confirm or otherwise and assess suspected pelvic mass(es)

86 When scanning the above patient, the sonographer should bear in mind:

— *What*: the sonographer should always ask the patient if the ovaries were left in situ during surgery. If the answer to the question is yes, efforts should be made to locate and assess the ovaries,

— *Why*: because the lady is of child-bearing age, unless the reason for her hysterectomy also involved the ovaries, gynaecologists tend to leave the ovaries of such patients in situ for hormonal needs.

87 Serous cystadenoma is the commonest benign tumour of the ovary seen in women aged 20–50 years old.

88 Serous cystadenoma is suggested by ultrasound findings of usually large (but may be small), thin-walled cysts, which may contain septa. About 30% are bilateral and may grow large enough to occupy most of the abdomen.

89 Serous cystadenocarcinoma presentations:

— cystic structure with or without internal material

— poorly defined walls

— considerable amount of solid tissue plus ascites.

♦ May be difficult to differentiate from the benign form of the cyst.

90 Complications of an ovarian mass include ovarian torsion, haemorrhage and rupture.

91 a] *Endometriosis* is the presence of endometrium in abnormal places outside the uterus (e.g. in the ovary, intestine, urinary bladder, pouch of Douglas or broad ligaments). These endometrial tissues respond to hormonal changes during the menstrual cycle, proliferating and bleeding throughout the cycle. Patients with endometriosis may present with chronic or acute-on-chronic pain. They may have 'chocolate' cysts, which persist without resolution and may increase in size.

Adenomyosis is a variant of endometriosis, in which the uterus is usually enlarged as a result of endometrial tissue in the myometrium. When the uterus is involved, it is known as adenomyomatosis.

b] Patients with endometriosis are usually in their twenties to thirties, nulliparous and infertile, while patients with adenomyosis are usually in their 40s, multiparous, might have had previous caesarean section, dilation and curettage (D&C) or elevated oestrogen levels.

c] Endometritis is an acute or chronic infective process of the endometrium.

d] Endometritis can arise following:

— instrumentation (e.g. D&C)

— insertion of an IUCD

— RPOC in the postpartum period

— premature rupture of the membranes (PROM)

— PID (with chronic PID, ascending venereal infection causes the endometritis).

e] There may be fluid in the endometrium, which may or may not be irregular in outline, may or may not have debris or internal echoes, and may have gas where there is a gas-forming organism. The uterus may be enlarged with an indistinct outline, with an endometrium that may or may not be thickened but with increased or decreased echogenicity. There may be an adnexal mass, pelvic fluid, pyosalpinx and tubovarian abscess.

♦ A normal ultrasound appearance may be seen in up to 75% of patients whose biopsy has revealed endometritis.

92 a] Endometrial cancer is a tumour of the uterine endometrial lining. It is most common in postmenopausal women with abnormal postmenopausal bleeding (PMB) and in premenopausal women with intramenstrual bleeding (IMB).

♦ It is the most common gynaecological malignant disease. It occurs in about 2.2% of women, greater than 70% occurring in women over 50 years old, 5% occurring in women under 40 years old.

b] Symptoms of endometrial cancer include PMB or IMB which is quoted as being seen in 90% of these women.

c] Ultrasound findings suggestive of endometrial cancer include an enlarged lobular uterus, hyper- or hypoechogenic uterine body, loss of or incomplete central hypoechoic line, and solid tissue arising from the endometrium and invading the myometrium and periuterine structures. The endometrial cavity often contains fluid (blood/pus) which is secondary to the obstruction of the normal drainage of the uterus.

♦ Poorly differentiated tumours of the endometrium (grades II and III) tend to be hypoechoic, whereas polypoid tumours are hyperechoic.

93 a] Teratomas account for approximately 10–15% of all ovarian neoplasms. They present most commonly during the reproductive years, are rare before puberty and rarely develop after the menopause.

b] In ovarian teratoma ultrasound is useful in:
— the evaluation of the patient following surgery
— the demonstration of residual tumour and metastases.

94 Cervical cancer can be indicated by:
— bulky cervix with irregular outline, possibly extending into the vagina or peritoneum
— a mass extending from the cervix to the pelvic sidewalls
— ureter entrapment and invasion leading to hydronephrosis
— invasion of the urinary bladder seen as an irregular mass effect on the bladder wall
— para-aortic node formation and liver metastases.

♦ Cervical cancer is a common genital tract malignancy in women, with the peak age for occurrence in the fourth decade.

95 Malignant ovarian teratoma can present on ultrasound as irregular masses with complex internal echoes. Both cystic and solid elements may be present and there may be acoustic shadowing. There may be ascites and metastatic deposits.

♦ Most patients with malignant ovarian teratoma (MOT) are in their twenties or thirties but MOT may also be seen in young children.

    c] Future ultrasound management may include:
- — cyst aspiration under ultrasound control if clinically indicated
- — assessing the kidneys to exclude hydronephrosis
- — excluding or confirming any associated abdominal/pelvic ascites
- — monitoring the patient's response to treatment(s).

◆ Asking the patient to empty her urinary bladder helps to confirm which of the cystic entities is the urinary bladder.

◆ Serous cystadenoma initially may look like a simple ovarian cyst, is usually unilocular with thin-walled septa and occasionally papillary projections. It may be bilateral and undergo malignant transformation into cystadenocarcinoma. Ascites may rarely be seen with it.

Obstetrics – 1st trimester

ANSWERS

1 Clinical indications for 1st trimester scanning include:
   — successful infertility treatment follow up
   — bleeding per vagina (PV) with or without pain in a patient who is aware that she is pregnant
   — irregular bleeding in a patient who is unaware that she is pregnant
   — dating the pregnancy accurately
   — excluding ectopic gestation
   — ascertaining any anatomical cause for hyperemesis in early pregnancy
   — planned triple test
   — confirming that the pregnancy is ongoing before and after cervical stitch
   — chorionic villus sampling (CVS) – before, during and immediately after
   — NT screening programme
   — preparation for termination of pregnancy (TOP).
      ◆ The GA will help the clinician to determine the choice of technique to use for TOP.

2 1st or 2nd trimester abdominal pain can be caused by:
   — ectopic gestation
   — abortion
   — large (> 5 cm) corpus luteal cyst
   — degeneration of a fibroid.

3 Urgent ultrasound scan should be performed in the 1st trimester for:
   — suspected ectopic gestation
   — suspected abortion
   — suspected molar pregnancy
   — low abdominal pain
   — abnormal PV bleed with or without pain
   — possible adnexal mass.

4 Bleeding in early pregnancy may be associated with anembryonic pregnancy, ectopic pregnancy, subchorionic haemorrhage, threatened abortion, inevitable abortion, incomplete abortion, leiomyomas, hydatidiform mole or gestational trophoblastic disease.

5 A full bladder is required for a TAS because:
   — it pushes the uterus out of the pelvis and thus it will not be overshadowed by the pubic bone
   — it displaces the bowel superiorly

b]

Person to consult	Reason for enquiry
Consultant obstetricians	To know what information they would want the
Consultant in charge of obstetric ultrasound in that hospital	patient to have with regard to the condition found via ultrasound To know the possible obstetric management for that condition
Antenatal clinic sister or counsellor/lead ward sister	As above, plus finding out the contact person and telephone number in that hospital
Other colleagues	Learning from their wealth of experience any useful tips and ideas. Since all the sonographers in that hospital will be using the leaflets, contents have to be agreed
Patients who have already been in this situation but who have subsequently had normal pregnancies and unaffected/normal child(ren)	From their experience they will provide you with the possible questions they would have wished to ask or information they would have wanted to be told at the time of the incident

c] Advantages of patient information leaflets include:
  — uniform information is given to all patients with a similar clinical condition in that hospital
  — hard copy, compact, basic information on the clinical condition is available for patients to refer to later
  — eliminating the problem of not conveying useful information about scan findings and the condition itself
  — names, addresses and telephone numbers of contact persons or support groups for the clinical condition, which could be useful for the couple, in the future
  — promoting good team spirit between the hospital staff.
  ◆ It is not uncommon that at the time of the incident, most of the information given by the staff is not taken in by the patient in view of feelings of shock, anger, frustration or the patient just wanting to get out of the hospital and go home first.

17 There is a limitation or inability of moving the transducer sufficiently to manipulate a lateral spine into an easier position for measurement.

18 An inaccurate CRL may be obtained if:
  — the yolk sac is included in the measurement
  — the longest length of the embryo/fetus is not measured
  — the measurement is taken with the embryo/fetus curled
  — the CRL is done after 14 weeks GA
  — the callipers are faulty.

19 The LMP is not always reliable for dating a pregnancy because:
  — date of LMP may not be known
  — the patient may have an irregular period
  — the patient may not have a 28-day cycle
  — the patient may have bled earlier in the pregnancy
  — the patient may have just stopped the oral contraceptive pill (OCP).

— the patient may have conceived on fertility treatment.

♦ For patients who conceive through fertility treatment, the pregnancy is dated using the known ovulation date or embryo transfer date.

20 Errors in establishing a LMP occur in women who become pregnant fewer than three menstrual cycles after ceasing use of the OCP because the interval between discontinuing the hormones and the onset of the ovulation is highly variable.

21 It is difficult to establish a LMP in:

— women who become pregnant fewer than three menstrual cycles after the last OCP

— women with oligomenorrhoea

— women who conceive while wearing an intrauterine contraceptive device (IUCD)

— women who become pregnant in the postpartum period before a normal menstrual cycle is re-established

— women who had bled earlier in pregnancy (slight uterine bleeding or spotting, which may occasionally occur after implantation of the blastocyst, may be incorrectly regarded as menstruation).

22 Measurement of gestational sac volume, gestational sac diameter or CRL, depending on the gestational age, will date a 1st trimester pregnancy.

23 a] The earliest ultrasound sign of pregnancy is the demonstration of a gestational sac (GS) within the uterus.

b] Endometrial thickening cannot be used to diagnose pregnancy because the same appearance can:

— be seen in a late phase of the menstrual cycle

— be seen in a very early intrauterine pregnancy, i.e. before the GS can be resolved

— be seen as a decidual reaction in association with ectopic pregnancy

— be confused with retained products of conception (RPOC) within the uterine cavity.

24 a] GSV is important:

— in the calculation of GA in women with uncertain dates when the CRL cannot be measured

— in the diagnosis of anembryonic pregnancy

— because any increase or decrease or no change in GSV over a period of time will help in confirming or otherwise the GA and continuity of the pregnancy.

b] GSV is the volume, whereby three measurements of the gestational sac are done and used, whereas the GSD is a single measurement of the widest diameter of the gestational sac.

♦ It has been suggested that failure of the gestational sac to increase in size by 75% in a week or no growth or abnormal growth (< 0.7 mm/day) is highly suggestive of anembryonic or abnormal pregnancy. With a GSV of 3 ml or a sac diameter of 25 mm, a fetal pole and fetal heartbeat (FHB) should be seen in a normally developing pregnancy. A GSD of 20 mm without a yolk sac (YS) or 25 mm without a fetal pole/embryo is generally associated with an anembryonic or abnormal gestation and it will eventually abort.

♦ GSV growth is very rapid between 5 and 10/40.

♦ Whether GSV or GSD is used will depend on departmental protocol.

should therefore be performed to rule out this possibility in patients receiving ovulatory drugs.

- ◆ Patients undergoing IVF programmes are said to be at a higher risk of heterotopic pregnancy, with an incidence as high as 1 in 100.
- ◆ Irregular vaginal bleeding occurs in 50–80% of ectopic pregnancies as a result of the sloughing of the decidual.
- ◆ Pseudogestational sac is seen in 10–20% of the cases.
- ◆ For unknown reasons, ectopic pregnancies occur less frequently in spring and summer.

39 Miscarriage is loss of pregnancy before 28 weeks GA.

40 Submucous fibroid may prevent pregnancy implantation or cause recurrent miscarriages.

41 Incompetent cervix may be caused by congenital absence of or damage to the circular layer of muscles that surround the internal os.

42 An incompetent cervix may be responsible for miscarriage in the 2nd trimester or for preterm labour.

43 Incompetent cervix may be suggested by the ultrasound findings of a cervix with a length of less than 2.5 cm and internal os width of more than 8 mm (normal range: length 2.5–10 cm, width 4 mm).

44 ● *Anembryonic pregnancy*: a gestational sac or trophoblastic ring of > 3 ml or a mean sac diameter of 25 mm without a fetal pole. There may be a discrepancy between the size of the sac and the uterine size. The sac may be too large or too small for the uterus.

● *Incomplete abortion*: an enlarged uterus, a partially expelled conceptus or placenta or an ill-defined gestational sac with internal echoes that are not specifically fetal will be seen.

● *Complete abortion*: a normal-sized or enlarged uterus (up to 2 weeks after the abortion) and a closed cervix with no ultrasound features of a pregnancy.

● *Threatened abortion*: a pregnancy with FHB, with a closed cervical os in the presence of vaginal bleeding. It is seen in about 25% of pregnancies and about 50% of such threatened abortions will invariably abort while the other half will progress successfully.

● *Inevitable abortion*: opened or widened cervical os, with the conceptus within or on its way out of the uterus. A fluid–fluid level may be present with the abortion.

● *Missed abortion*: an intrauterine gestational sac with a fetal pole but without a fetal heartbeat, or a crumpled sac and embryo/fetus, mostly occurring between 6 and 14/40.

● *Septic abortion*: an enlarged uterus with increased endometrial echoes. Shadowing from retained bony fragments of conception following an attempted abortion, or from gas-forming organisms if due to infection, may be seen.

● The use of an ultrasound scan in the management of an abortion can be to confirm that the pregnancy is ongoing, or to help the patients come to terms with the inevitability of their situation, or to exclude products of conception. Good communication skills are essential in the sonographer.

45 a] Clinical presentation of a hydatidiform mole may include:
— no periods

    — uterus bigger than the expected dates
    — a lot of nausea or vomiting
    — irregular bleeding which may contain fluid-filled cysts or vesicular tissue
    — symptoms suggestive of miscarriage between 8 and 16/40
    — thyrotoxicosis
    — Pre-eclampsia.

b]
- *Complete mole*: this is caused by a sperm fusing with an egg which has no genetic material (DNA). Such a fertilized egg implanting in the uterus grows only the trophoblast (chorion).
  - It is possible to have a twin pregnancy in which a normal fetus has as the twin a complete mole.
- *Partial mole*: this is caused when two sperm fertilize a normal egg. There is too much genetic material and an embryo/fetus may or may not be present. Such an embryo/fetus does not develop and the placenta outgrows it.
  - It is important that a partial mole is diagnosed so that the appropriate treatment can be given following dilation and curettage (D&C).
- *Invasive mole*: where the trophoblast of a complete mole spreads outside the uterus with a high risk of death from severe haemorrhage as the invasive molar villi may embolize in the lung and brain.
- *Choriocarcinoma*: where the trophoblast invades and spreads widely. Distant metastases are common in the lungs, liver, brain, gastrointestinal tract (GIT), kidneys and pelvic organs. This may follow a complete mole and rarely may follow a normal pregnancy, miscarriage or TOP. It is a rare malignancy with a quoted incidence of 1 in 30 000 pregnancies.

c] No fetus will be seen on ultrasound in a complete mole; in a partial mole a GS may be seen with a growth-retarded fetus, no normal placenta or rather an excessive-in-size placenta with many cystic spaces randomly distributed within it (differential diagnoses – missed or incomplete abortion).

d] Follow-up diagnostic tests in choriocarcinoma include X-ray, CT or MRI, Duplex and colour-flow Doppler in order to detect choriocarcinoma or an invasive mole and assess the extent of the spread.

e] Pregnancy during the time of follow up may mimic the high levels of hCG which are seen when the mole is recurring, thus making detection of recurrence difficult.

f] Contraceptive pills may prolong the life of the remaining mole cells.

g] For a woman who has had one mole the chances of having another mole have been quoted as 1 in 80. For a woman who has had two molar pregnancies the chances for a third have been quoted as 1 in 6.
  - Previous history of molar pregnancy, Asian ancestry and increasing maternal age may all render a woman at greater risk of molar pregnancy.

h] It has been suggested that there is no greater risk of abnormal babies in women who have had chemotherapy.

46 A 1st trimester gravid uterus containing an anembryonic gestational sac, often surrounded by a thick ring of densely echogenic trophoblastic tissue, may progress to hydatidiform mole.

63 Technical problems during CVS include inability to obtain enough villus material and the presence of vaginal infection (if the transcervical route is used).

64 CVS is not recommended in multiple pregnancy because there is no guarantee that both placentas have been sampled, especially where it is not known if there is one single placenta or there are two placentas located one next to the other.

65 • Direct preparation:
  — result known within 48 hours
  — no contamination from the decidua cells, thus no false result.
 • Culture preparation:
  — more mitoses, thus more accurate in detecting chromosomal changes. It does however, take 7–10 days to get the result.
 ◆ It is advisable to employ both techniques.

66 Disadvantages of direct preparation:
  — direct preparation of the chorionic villi produces fewer mitoses than culture and thus may not be able to detect minor chromosomal changes (villus culture is advisable as well)
  — since the sample being used is from the placenta (trophoblast), it may not demonstrate the same karyotype as the fetus
  — there may be contamination from overgrown maternal cells and thus a false result.

67 Pregnancy loss following CVS is quoted as 1–4% (1% in trained operator and expert hands).

68 CVS may lead to limb deformity through hypoperfusion, embolization or release of vasoactive substances. These are all related to trauma during the procedure. The risks can be eliminated by trained operators performing CVS only after 11/40 GA and under ultrasound control.
 ◆ Operators are mostly obstetricians and gynaecologists.

69 • Nuchal thickness (NT) is the subcutaneous translucency between the skin and soft tissue overlying the cervical spine.
 • Measurement of NT:
  — obtain a sagittal section of the fetus with the fetus in a neutral position, i.e. without flexing or hyperextension of the neck, which decreases or increases the measurement.
  — magnify the image on the TV monitor such that the fetus occupies at least 75% of the image
  — measure the subcutaneous translucency between the skin and soft tissue overlying the cervical spine. This measurement should not include the amnion so care must be taken to distinguish between the fetal skin and the amnion. The callipers are placed as shown in the diagram in Fig. A4.69
  — at least two or three measurements should be taken but the maximum thickness is to be recorded.
 ◆ Where the umbilical cord is round the fetal neck, it produces an indentation in the nuchal membrane, making the translucency larger above, rather than below the cord.
 ◆ NT measurement is done with a CRL of 45 mm–84 mm or GA of 11/40 – 13^{+6}/40.

A4.69

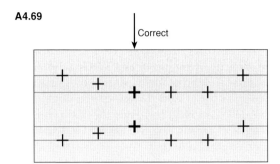

- ◆ Cord around the fetal neck is seen in 5–10% of cases where there is discrepancy between the NT measurement below and above the cord. To calculate the risk, the smaller of the two measurements is used i.e. the measurement below the cord.
70 • Nuchal thickness is described in Answer 69 above; it is measured in the 1st trimester and in a sagittal section.
   • Nuchal fold (NF) is measured in the 2nd trimester, on a suboccipitobregmatic view demonstrating the midline, cerebellum and cisterna magna. The measurement is taken from the outer table of the occiput to the outer border of the skin.
   ◆ The normal range of NF measurement is ≤ 6 mm at 18–20 weeks GA. A greater value may indicate Down's syndrome.
71 The background risk is calculated using the maternal age, gestational age and previous history of chromosomal defects multiplied by a series of factors which depend on the results of a series of screening tests carried out during the course of that pregnancy.
72 Sequential screening is a process whereby every time a test is carried out, the background risk is multiplied by the test factor to calculate a new risk which then becomes the background risk for the next test.
73 a] The older the mother the higher the risk for trisomy.
   b] The earlier the GA the higher the risk for trisomy. Fetuses with chromosomal defects are more likely to die in utero than normal fetuses therefore the risk decreases with GA.
   c] If a woman has had a previous fetus or baby with trisomy 21, the risk for trisomy 21 in her current pregnancy is quoted as being three times the background risk.
74 a] The higher the NT measurement, the higher the risk for trisomies.
   b] The higher the maternal serum hCG, the higher the risk for trisomy 21.
   c] The lower the maternal serum PAPP-A, the higher the risk for trisomy 21.
75 NT measurement normally increases with GA and thus CRL.
   ◆ It has been observed that the 95th centile was 2.2 mm for CRL of 38 mm and 2.8 mm for a CRL of 84 mm. However, the 99th centile did not change significantly with CRL and was approximately 3.5 mm (see Further reading)
76 One fetus or child with a NTD gives a 1 in 20 chance of recurrence but this reduces to 1 in 10 if the woman has already had two fetuses or children with NTD.

77 In monochorionic (MC) pregnancy, there is no extension of the placenta into the membrane and thus the junction of the placenta and the intertwin membrane forms a T sign. In dichorionic (DC) pregnancy, there is an extension of the placenta into the base of the intertwin membrane, forming the lambda sign (λ).

78 DZ twins show marked racial differences; for example in Caucasians, the incidence is 1 in 80 deliveries but in West Africa, especially among the Yoruba tribe in Nigeria, the incidence is 1 in 20 deliveries, the rate increasing with maternal age until 39 years of age when it declines. Other factors which affect DZ twinning include parity, height and weight. There is also familial tendency which is inherited through the maternal line.

♦ It has been suggested that since the Yoruba tribe eats a variety of yam that contains substances with oestrogen-like properties, this may induce ovulation through the secretion of high follicle stimulating hormone (FSH) levels.

Incidence of MZ twins is about the same in all populations – 3–5% per 1000 births. It is less likely to be affected by maternal age.

79

MZ twins	DZ twins
Develop from one ovum	Develop from two ova
Begin in the blastocyst stage around the end of the 1st week and result from division of the inner cell mass or embyroblast into two embryonic primordia	Begin as two separate zygotes
Same sex	Not necessarily the same sex
Genetically identical	Genetically no more identical than two siblings from the same parents

Physical differences between MZ twins at birth are environmentally induced (e.g. due to twin–twin transfusion syndrome).

80 The phenomenon of conjoined twins is seen in MZ twins when the embryoblast or embryonic disc does not divide completely. Incidence has been quoted as about 1 in 40 of MZ pregnancies.

81 In conjoined twins ultrasound is used to:
— date the pregnancy accurately
— establish the type of conjoined twins, i.e. the organs shared and to what extent
— monitor their growth in utero.

82 Triplets can develop from:
— two ova: a singleton from one ovum and a set of MZ (genetically identical) twins from the other ovum
— three separate ova: the triplets may or may not be of the same sex. Genetically they will be no more identical than siblings from the same parents.

83 Early diagnosis of twins is important:
— to give an accurate GA as preterm delivery may be contemplated later
— to determine the chorionicity of twins especially for MZ/MC twins which have the highest perinatal morbidity and mortality due to the presence of vascular anastomoses within the chorionic plate
— in view of a greater frequency and earlier onset of complications

 — to enable appropriate counselling and planning of future care (e.g. close monitoring of ongoing pregnancy).

84 Chorionicity and amnionicity data are important in differentiating IUGR and if selective feticide is considered.

 ◆ In MC twins there is a risk that embolization of thromboplastins from the dead twin can affect the surviving twin.

 ◆ MC twins are associated with an increased risk of prematurity, fetal malformations, twin–twin transfusion syndrome (TTTS) and consequent increased perinatal morbidity and mortality.

85 Vanishing twin syndrome occurs when twins have been diagnosed by ultrasound showing two fetuses, each with FHB at the 1st trimester, but it ends in a singleton at delivery.

 ◆ PV bleed may occur and vanishing twin incidence is estimated at 20% of twin pregnancies diagnosed at the 1st trimester scan.

86 Ultrasound artefacts that may mimic twins include retromembranous haematomas, chorioamniotic separation, occasional YS, bicornuate uterus and empty second sac.

87

A4.87

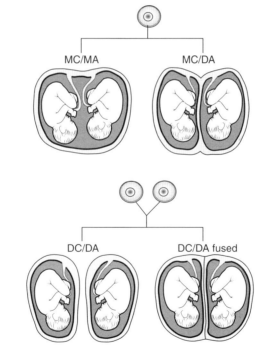

 ◆ Twins do not necessarily lie in the same direction.

 ◆ 80% of twins are DZ and 20% are MZ.

 ◆ 80% of MZ twins have dichorionic placentas and 20% have a monochorionic placenta.

 ◆ DZ twins always have two placentas and thus different circulations.

88 The amniotic sac membrane surrounds the amniotic fluid. It is often seen in the 1st trimester but fuses with the chorion by 12–15/40. In multiple pregnancy, it is

seen to separate gestational sacs that are not monoamniotic (MA) from late on in the 1st trimester.

89 In MZ twins the amniotic sac membrane has two components; in DZ twins the membrane is thicker and has four components. In MZ twins there is therefore the possibility of many associated anomalies, for example conjoined twins, polyhydramnios, locking twins, asymmetrical growth and entangled cord. Details of the amniotic sac membrane should be recorded because the type of twin may influence obstetrics management of the pregnancy, for example in some departments, MC twins are scanned at 20, 24, 28, 32 and 36 weeks GA and DC twins are scanned at 20, 28, 32 and 36 weeks GA routinely.

90 • In dichorionic/diamniotic (DA) twins, there is a thick membrane made up of two chorionic and two amniotic layers which separates the gestational sacs.
   • In MC/DA twins the membranes between the gestational sacs are very thin (two amniotic layers only) but a thick chorion surrounds the twins and there is one placenta.
   • In MC/MA twins – which are rare – a single chorion and amnion surrounds the twins and it is not possible to see a membrane between them on ultrasound. There is one placenta.
   ◆ It has been suggested that DC membranes have a mean thickness of 2.4 mm and a lambda sign (λ) is seen at the base of the septum dividing the twins near the placenta. A thin membrane, i.e. thickness < 2 mm (mean 1.4 mm), is suggestive of a monochorion.

91 Features of DZ twins on ultrasound include:
   — separate placenta sites
   — different fetal gender
   — very thick dividing membrane with four components, i.e. two amnions and two chorions (this is a particularly reliable guide in the 1st and 2nd trimester).

92 Reasons for scanning multiple pregnancy include:
   — diagnosing multiple pregnancy and dating accurately
   — determining chorionicity
   — detection of fetal abnormality
   — detection of discordant growth
   — monitoring of fetal growth.

93 Zygote division and resulting twin type:
   — a zygote that divides 4 days after fertilization results in DC/DA gestation
   — a zygote that divides between 4 and 8 days after fertilization results in MC/DA gestation
   — a zygote that divides 8 days after fertilization results in MC/MA gestation
   — division of the embryonic disc 13 days or more after conception results in conjoined twins.

94 It is best to determine chorionicity between 9 and 10 weeks GA because the amnion is not clearly seen by the TVS until 8/40.

95 Each twin has the CRL and the NT measured as for a singleton. In DC twins the individual NT measurement for each twin is combined with the maternal age and the risk for trisomies is calculated for that particular twin. There will thus be two

risk factors for DC twins but in MC twins, because they are identical, the greater NT measurement is combined with the maternal age and the risk for trisomies is calculated for both twins. There is thus only one risk factor for MC twins.

♦ As with singleton pregnancies, increased NT may be a marker of cardiac or other defects or a marker of TTTS in MC twins.

♦ In MC twins increased NT may also be a marker of TTTS.

96 a] The ultrasound appearances are of an anteverted uterus that appears normal in size with a thick endometrium (measurement not indicated). No intrauterine gestational sac (IUGS) was demonstrated. Within the cavity is a hyperechoic area surrounded by a hypoechoic area, possibly representing some fluid.

b] Ultrasound appearances are suggestive of incomplete abortion with possible retained products of conception (RPOC).

97 a] The ultrasound appearances are of a bulky uterus measuring $106 \times 86 \times 85$ mm. No IUGS was demonstrated. A rather typical snowstorm appearance is demonstrated.

b] This is possibly a hydatidiform mole (complete mole).

♦ Differential diagnosis will be a missed abortion with hydropic degeneration or degenerating fibroid but this will not have the same clinical presentation.

♦ Very rarely in a twin pregnancy, a normal fetus may be seen along with a mole.

♦ Hydatidiform mole occurrence is quoted as 1 in 300 in Asians but 1 in 3000 in Caucasians.

c]

Location	Reason for investigation
Ovaries	For large cysts (called theca lutein cysts) which are follicles that have been stimulated because of increased hCG
Liver	For metastases which are usually seen with choriocarcinoma

Theca lutein cysts are seen in 40% of moles.

d] Future ultrasound management would involve scanning early in any subsequent pregnancy in order to rule out another mole.

♦ Mole confirmed at D&C.

98 a] In Fig. 4.98a three gestational sacs are seen within the uterus. Yolk sacs, fetal poles and FHB were reported as seen. In Fig. 4.98b there are two gestational sacs. Sac 1 has two yolk sacs and fetal poles, while sac 2 has a single fetal pole. Both ladies are carrying a set of triplets each.

b] The triplets in Fig. 4.98a are non-identical, each coming from three different ova, whereas in Fig. 4.98b there is a set of MC twins (i.e. from the same ovum) and the third embryo is from a separate ovum.

c] The triplets in Fig 4.98b are at a higher risk because of the MC twins.

d] Future ultrasound management:

— should the fetocide option be considered in order to reduce the triplets to twins, it will be under ultrasound monitor

— assessing the fetal anatomy of the triplets

— growth monitoring of the triplets.

103 a] The ultrasound appearances are of an anteverted uterus which appeared to be normal in size. No intrauterine gestational sac was demonstrated. Some mixed echo fluid was seen in the cavity, especially in the cervical area.

    b] Differential diagnosis is of an ongoing abortion which is not complete.

    c] The role of ultrasound is to assess the uterus and any ultrasound-identifiable explanation for the PV bleed. The sonographer will need to confirm to the patient the pregnancy loss and this may help her to come to terms with it.
   - The ultrasound findings will help the clinicians to determine if there is any need for D&C.

104 a] The ultrasound appearances are of an anteverted uterus seen with an intrauterine gestational sac, yolk sac, fetal pole and FHB. Fetal pole appears too small to be measured. GSV/GSD measurements were not included.

    b] The sonographer should also comment on the state of the cervix.

    c] The diagnosis is of threatened abortion.

    d] The role of ultrasound is to confirm and date the pregnancy, check the state of the patient's cervix, assess fetal anatomy and growth in line with departmental protocol.

    e] The pregnancy is ≥ 5 weeks but < 7 weeks (this is because there is a FHB, YS, fetal pole but no measurable CRL as yet). Rescanning the lady in 2–3 weeks from that date (depending on departmental protocol) will reconfirm if the pregnancy is ongoing and a measurable CRL will be obtainable by then.

105 a] The most significant ultrasound finding is a huge cystic structure in the fetal abdomen.

    b] This cystic structure could originate from the urinary tract or, less likely, from the GIT.

    c] If the cystic structure continues to grow, the abdominal organs and chest will be compressed. This will affect lung development.

106 a] Fig. 4.106a shows a TAS while Fig. 4.106b shows a TVS. Both demonstrate a retroverted uterus with an intrauterine gestational sac, yolk sac and fetal pole with FHB. CRL = 20 mm = dates.

    b] Differential diagnosis is of a threatened abortion.

    c] The uterine fundus and the upper part of the cavity line may be difficult to visualize because the ultrasound beam may not be at a right angle to it. Further filling the bladder will possibly displace the uterus further away from the probe.
   - Retroverted uterus is more common after pregnancy and is noted in about 33% of women.
   - Vaginal bleeding is said to occur in one-third of all pregnancies. About 50% of pregnancies experiencing bleeding will ultimately abort spontaneously. Demonstrating the FHB in a patient who is bleeding reduces the risk of spontaneous abortion from about 40–50% to 1.3–2.6% depending on the GA when the fetal heart is first imaged.
   - Some pregnant women experience PV bleed following intercourse.

107 a] The ultrasound appearances are of an anteverted uterus with an 8.8 mm hyperechoic endometrium. No IUGS was demonstrated. The right ovary had a

normal echopattern and there is a 15 mm corpus luteal cyst in the left ovary. In the right adnexus was a gestational sac and fetal pole with FHB. No obvious free fluid was demonstrated in the POD or around the gestational sac.

b] Differential diagnosis is of a right ectopic pregnancy, confirmed by the FHB.

c] If the pregnancy is a tubal pregnancy and the fallopian tube cannot be saved, this lady will need some form of assisted reproduction technique in conceiving subsequently.

- Surgery confirmed an unruptured right tubal pregnancy.
- The major clinical concern following an ectopic pregnancy is poor reproductive performance. Only about half of the patients will conceive again, with a risk of a second ectopic pregnancy of 10–20%.

108 a] The ultrasound appearances are of an anteverted uterus with a thickened endometrium measuring 15 mm. The left ovary was 38×32 mm and had a normal echopattern. On the right was a GS, YS, fetal pole but no FHB. CRL = 16 mm = 8/40. No free fluid was demonstrated in the POD or surrounding the GS. The right ovary was not demonstrated separately from this GS.

b] The differential diagnoses include right ovarian pregnancy, tubal pregnancy or abdominal pregnancy.

c] The progesterone-only pill makes the cervical mucus hostile to the sperm and makes the endometrium secretive, preventing implantation of the blastocyst.

- Women on the progesterone-only pill can still ovulate but occasionally they can stop ovulating completely.
- Women on this type of pill are at a higher risk of an ectopic pregnancy.

d] Factors leading to pregnancy while on the pill

Combined oral contraceptive pill	Progesterone-only pill
Certain antibiotics	Vomiting the pill
Certain drugs which induce liver enzymes so that the pill does not work	Severe diarrhoea
Missing the 12-hour window	Missing the 3-hour window

Missing the combined pill at the beginning of the packet is more dangerous in terms of getting pregnant than at the end.

109 Asking the mother to cough or to lie on her side might bring about a change in fetal position or asking the mother to bend her knees with the soles of her feet firm on the couch, lifting up her hips and gently shaking her hips might encourage the fetus to move and change position. If all fails, send the woman for a walk and scan some minutes later.

110 a] Ultrasound shows an intrauterine gestational sac with a single fetus. CRL was reported to be = GA by LMP and FHB and movements were reported as seen. The NT is 7.1 mm, there is generalized oedema and bilateral pleural effusion.

b] Differential diagnosis is of cystic hygroma (non-septated) and bilateral pleural effusion.

c] Future ultrasound management should include (depending on patient's wishes and the clinician):

— preterm labour
— large or small for dates
— placenta localization
— fetal weight estimate
— suspected intrauterine death (IUD)
— oligo- or polyhydramnios
— follow up of fetuses:
  • with known structural abnormalities
  • following in utero therapeutic treatments (e.g. post stent insertion) and monitoring.

4 a] Women susceptible to preterm labour and delivery include those:
— who have had a previous preterm baby
— with cervical incompetence
— with multiple pregnancy
— with maternal diabetes mellitus
— with polyhydramnios
— with bacterial vaginosis.

b] Clinical indications for ultrasound of the cervix:
— to confirm or refute an incompetent cervix in a woman who is symptomatic or non-symptomatic (e.g. as in the preterm risk assessment screening test)
— in patients with preterm labour
— in patients with 2nd or 3rd trimester polyhydramnios.
  ◆ Ultrasound can be used in guiding the position of the cervical cerclage (ligature).
  ◆ Shirodkar and McDonald sutures are techniques used in cervical cerclage.

c] Assessing the cervix

Method	Advantage	Disadvantage	Limitations
Translabial	Can be used where TVS or internal examination is contraindicated[a] Useful in emergency situations as empty urinary bladder is required	None	Entire cervical canal may not be visualized in a small percentage of patients
TAS	Non-threatening to patients with confirmed incompetent cervix or preterm labour	Full urinary bladder required and as such in emergency situations it may not be practicable	A dilated cervix can be masked by an overfilled urinary bladder Cervical length can be falsely increased Acoustic shadows from fetal parts, especially fetal head later in pregnancy, can make cervical assessment difficult May be difficult in obese patients Non-uniform urinary bladder volume may cause variations in measurement obtained

Assessing the cervix – *contd.*

Method	Advantage	Disadvantage	Limitations
TVS	Reproducible method More accurate way of assessing the cervix Use of higher frequency probes means better resolution Useful in obese patients Empty urinary bladder requirement is an advantage, especially in emergency situations	Limited field of view where the probe has < 90° scanning angle	Contraindicated in a few women[b]

TAS, transabdominal scan; TVS, transvaginal scan.

[a] TVS or internal examination is contraindicated where the patient has vaginismus, there is the possibility of uterine infection or the membrane is already ruptured.

[b] TVS may increase the risk of amnionitis in women with ruptured membranes, induce PV bleed in women with placenta praevia and cause contractions in women with preterm labour.

    d] In addition to Answer 34, Chapter 3 (p. 249), TVS assessment of the cervix should include the following:

      — the transvaginal (TV) probe should be carefully positioned in the anterior fornix of the vagina

      — a sagittal view of the cervix and cervical canal should be obtained

      — the triangular area of the external os and the echogenic V-shaped notch at the internal os should be identified and the distance between them measured

      — the best and shortest cervical measurement of the three measurements taken over a period of about 3 minutes should be recorded

      — the cervical image should be magnified to occupy at least 75% of the screen.

      ♦ It is not uncommon to notice changes in the cervix in the course of the examination; this is due to contractions and is seen in up to 1% of patients.

      ♦ Care must be taken to avoid undue pressure on the cervix as this will cause false elongation.

      ♦ In one centre in the UK, a cervical length of < 15 mm in a singleton pregnancy, or < 20 mm in a multiple pregnancy at 23/40, is considered to be a high risk for preterm delivery. Such women are referred to the obstetrician for counselling and follow up.

    e] In cervix assessment, note:

      — cervical length measurement

      — any cervical funnelling

      — cervical canal dilatation.

      ♦ Ultrasound findings of the cervix should be interpreted bearing in mind the GA of the pregnancy at the time of the scan as the same appearance may have different meanings at different gestational ages.

    f] Risks associated with cervical cerclage include infection, rupturing of the membrane and induction of labour.

14 In utero diagnostic techniques include:
   — CVS
   — amniocentesis
   — cordocentesis
   — ultrasound examination
   — fetoscopy, fetal skin or liver biopsy
   — X-ray from 10/40 for prenatal diagnosis of skeletal dysplasia (best at 20/40)
   — computed tomography (CT)
   — magnetic resonance imaging (MRI).

15 Ultrasound scan in the 2nd or 3rd trimester should record the number of fetuses, the presence or absence of cardiac activity, fetal presentation, placenta location (especially in relation to the internal os), fetal measurement femur length (FL), BPD, AC, HC) and estimate of the amniotic fluid volume.
   ◆ In many hospitals, the amniotic fluid is assessed subjectively, except in cases of oligo- or polyhydramnios.

16 Scan of a multiple pregnancy should record the information detailed in Answer 15 above plus sac number, fetal gender if seen (depending on departmental protocol) comparison of fetal size and chorionicity if not documented before. A diagrammatic representation of fetal presentation is useful (see Fig. A5.16).

A5.16

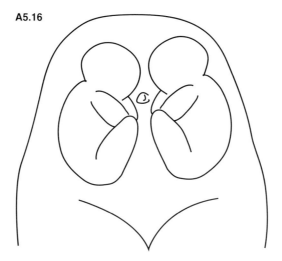

17 a] Depending on departmental protocol, FL, BPD, HC and AC should be measured after 14 weeks.
   b] Charts 1 and 2 in the Appendix (pp 415, 416) show, using FL as an example, the differences between dating and growth charts.
   ◆ Please note that in the chart used for dating, length of gestation is on the X axis but it is on the Y axis for the growth chart.
   c] A *plotted chart* is one in which the AC or HC is measured directly. In a *derived chart* (e.g. of AC), the transverse and anteroposterior (AP) measurements of the fetal abdomen are used to calculate the measurements. For the derived HC chart, the BPD and occipitofrontal diameter (OFD) are used to calculate the HC.

It is not uncommon for a department to state which method should be used in measuring the HC or AC as well as providing an appropriate chart for this in their protocol, although there may be another type of chart available for use if and when required.

18 a] An ultrasound 'soft marker' is an ultrasound-identifiable variation in an anatomical feature that may or may not be an indication for an underlying fetal chromosomal abnormality.

b] An ultrasound soft marker such as duodenal atresia (double bubble) is considered indicative of possible underlying fetal chromosomal abnormality and further invasive tests may need to be performed to rule this out. However, other soft markers such as isolated choroid plexus cyst (ICPC) may or may not be further investigated.

♦ It is important for the sonographer to be familiar with the soft markers indicated in the departmental protocols. Effort should be made to exclude any structural abnormality.

♦ Asking for a second opinion from a colleague is in the best interests of the patient and ought not be seen as an indication of incompetency.

♦ In many departments, finding any two soft markers is a clinical reason for further fetal assessment with or without invasive testing.

♦ Invasive testing will be influenced by the patient's decision for or against it.

c] Soft markers include: duodenal atresia, overlapping fingers, rockerbottom feet, choroid plexus cyst (CPC), ICPC, talipes, 'golf ball', renal pelvis dilatation > 5 mm, nuchal fold (NF) > 6 mm at the anomaly scan, and echogenic bowels.

d] With a FMU it may be easier to follow up cases and pregnancy outcome. The FMU may also act as an external system of quality assurance in auditing. Additionally, it is easier to refer patients to the FMU because of the good rapport between the two departments.

e] Fetal abnormalities should be notified to the Congenital Malformation Register Office for that region of the UK.

f] Records are currently required by law to be kept for a specific number of years. Different hospitals also have protocols for how long their ultrasound records will be kept.

♦ This will also be influenced by individual hospital policy on recording ultrasound examinations and on storing ultrasound records, especially the hard copy.

g] For those performing obstetric ultrasound scans, the basic requirements are governed by the various codes of conduct relating to their own professional bodies, as advocated by, for example, the College of Radiographers.

h] The United Kingdom Association of Sonographers (UKAS) *Guidelines for professional working standards – ultrasound practice* (1996) has identified the following medicolegal issues:

— in all circumstances, sonographers will be legally accountable for their professional actions including reporting

— the ultrasound report is a public document and part of the hospital medical records, together with any images which may accompany it. These images where recorded may be used to support, or refute, the content of the report.

28

Organ	Position	Ultrasound appearance
Stomach	Left side, below the diaphragm	Hypoechoic, variable size depending on the time of last fetal swallowing
Spleen	Left side, below the diaphragm	Homogenous hyperechoic texture
Liver	Right side, below the diaphragm	Homogenous hyperechoic texture
Gall bladder	Right side	Hypoechoic
Kidneys	Both sides in the posterior abdomen	Hyperechoic with hypoechoic renal pelvis paraspinal
Urinary bladder	Midline in the pelvis	Round hypoechoic structure between the pelvic bones
Cord insertion	In the central abdominal wall	Usually three vessels, i.e. one vein and two arteries, but may be two vessels, i.e.one artery and one vein in some fetuses
Large bowel	In the periphery of the abdomen	Hypoechoic to hyperechoic and less than 7 mm in diameter
Small bowel	Central in the lower abdomen	Same as large bowel

29 UKAS recommends that the following fetal structures be checked:
- Fetal head: both cerebral lateral ventricles including each choroid plexus posterior fossa, nuchal area
- Facial views: profile, coronal views of the face and lips
- Thorax: chest contents, 4-chamber view of the heart and connecting vessels
- Abdomen: stomach, diaphragm, abdominal wall, kidneys, renal pelves, urinary bladder, cord insertion and number of vessels in the cord
- Others:
  — spine and its covering in longitudinal and transverse planes
  — 12 long bones, two hands and feet
  — genitalia if clinically relevant
  — fetal movements, heart and pulsation
  — amniotic fluid volume
  — placenta appearance and site relative to the internal cervical os.
- UKAS recommends that the sonographer be able to measure following fetal structures: BPD, AC, HC, FL, cerebral ventricles, limb lengths, NF, orbital diameters, renal and pelvic diameters.

30 a] The fetal face should be scanned in the sagittal plane to check the fetal face profile, in the coronal plane to check the fetal lips and nose, and in the transverse plane to check for hyper- or hypotelorism by measuring the orbital distance.

b] Fetal facial structures should be checked because an abnormality of the face can be a subtle indication of a chromosomal abnormality.

c] Proboscis is an ultrasound-recognizable mass that can arise from the fetal face.

31 a] Planes for examining the normal fetal spine

Section	Normal ultrasound appearance
Transverse	U shape
Sagittal	Gentle curve forward in the thoracic area, skin covering and sacral up-sweep
Coronal	Both posterior elements; the spinal cord may be seen within the spinal canal and can be traced to about the level of L1

See Question 54 in Chapter 1, Fig. 1.54b–e, 1.54g, 1.54h, 1.54k and 1.54l (pp 12–14).

b] • Spinal abnormalities best seen in coronal and sagittal section:
— scoliosis
— hemivertebrae
— location of a spinal defect
— extent of a spinal defect, i.e. how many vertebrae are involved and the skin integrity overlying the defect.
• Spinal abnormality best seen in transverse section: small spinal defect.

32 In LS the fetal cervical spine is a wine-glass shape (see Question 54 in Chapter 1, Fig. 1.54b, p. 12).

33 There are three ossification centres in the fetal spine: one for the vertebral body and the other two for the lateral processes which form the spinal canal. On the transverse section the three ossification centres form a triangle, on the coronal section the two ossification centres form two sets of parallel dots which taper down to a point in the sacrum, and on the LS two parallel white lines composed of echoes represent the vertebrae.

34 a] Spina bifida is a bony defect in the spine.
b] Ultrasound appearances of spina bifida include:
— banana-shaped cerebellum rather than the dumb-bell shape
— lemon-shaped head rather than the rugby-ball shape, i.e. blunting of the sinciput
— the three ossification centres form a V shape on transverse section instead of the normal U shape and strands of nervous tissue or discrete sac of meningocele may be seen
— a break in the skin covering may be seen on longitudinal section (if it is an open spina bifida)
— dilated cerebral ventricles in cases of spina bifida with hydrocephalus which is diagnosed by an increased anterior ventricular hemisphere ratio (AVHR).
c] Spina bifida affected fetuses are able to move their limbs in utero because the nerves are not fully developed in utero and are not yet exposed to air. The nervous disturbance is only manifested when exposed to air following delivery.
d] Spina bifida and anencephaly are both NTDs. However, defective closure at the upper (cephalic) end causes anencephaly, while that of the lower (caudal) end causes spina bifida.

e] Incidence of NTD varies geographically, for example:

Country	Incidence
Africa, Canada, Japan, Mongolia and USA	1:1000 births
South-east England	3:1000 births
West of Scotland	5:1000 births
South Wales	7.6:1000 births
Northern Ireland	8.6:1000 births
Eire	1:100 births

   ♦ It has been suggested that:
      — NTD occurs in 4.9% of all abortions, therefore about 16:1000 of all
         conceptions are affected
      — there is an increased frequency in lower social class and winter-born
         children
      — most NTDs are multifactorial but some are secondary to teratogenic
         influences (e.g. sodium valproate and maternal diabetes mellitus).
35 Myelomeningocele is indicated on ultrasound by:
   — V-shaped spine on transverse section instead of the U shape
   — presence of meningocele sac plus strands of nervous tissue
   — break in the skin coverage on the longitudinal section
   — separation of the line of ossification centres.
36 Encephalocele has no septa, there will be a bony defect in the skull and it may
   contain solid matter (i.e. brain), whereas cystic hygroma may have septa, there
   will be no bony defect in the skull and it is cystic. Cystic hygroma is often
   associated with chromosomal abnormalities such as Turner's syndrome and
   trisomies 21, 18 and 13.
37 Fetal heart, lungs, ribs and the diaphragm are the thoracic structures to check.
38 a] On ultrasound normal fetal lungs appear as two homogeneous echogenic
      structures which surround the heart and fill the chest cavity.
   b] Cystic adenomatoid malformation can make the fetal lungs appear more
      echogenic.
39 a] Brain structures to be checked at the anomaly scan include midline echo,
      cavum septum pellucidum, thalami, cerebellum, cisterna magna, choroid
      plexus and lateral ventricles.
   b] A normal cavum septum pellucidum excludes agenesis of corpus callosum and
      lobar holoprosencephaly.
   c] Normal ventricular measurement excludes ventriculomegaly and
      hydrocephalus.
   d] Normal cerebellum and cisterna magna exclude spina bifida, Dandy–Walker
      syndrome, cerebellar hypoplasia, enlarged cisterna magna, Arnold–Chiari
      malformation (which is caused by spina bifida) and NTD.
   e] The diameter of the cisterna magna normally measures 4–10 mm.
   f] Mild ventriculomegaly is indicated by an atrial width of 10–15 mm (≥ 11 mm is
      considered abnormal at any GA).
   g] The fetal cisterna magna is difficult to identify in Arnold–Chiari malformation.

h] The 4th ventricle can be seen when it is enlarged. It is normally anterior to the cerebellum.

i] Enlarged AVHR, flattened and thin choroid plexus or dangling choroid plexus, and opposed medial walls of the lateral ventricles are indicative of ventriculomegaly.

♦ Cavum septum pellucidum should be one-third of the way from the sinciput to the occiput.

♦ Between 13 and 22 weeks GA, BPD has an accuracy of 5–10 days and up to 4 weeks after a GA of 30 weeks.

♦ Normally, the choroid plexus should fill the lateral ventricles.

♦ In cases of suspected or confirmed ventriculomegaly, it is essential that the structures of the brain (especially those of the posterior fossa and midline) are evaluated to confirm how many ventricles are involved and to confirm or otherwise if the dilatation is asymmetrical or symmetrical. Atrial measurements should be noted and other structural abnormalities excluded.

♦ Intraventricular bleed or infection (e.g. CMV, parvovirus) has been suggested to cause symmetrically dilated ventricles with echogenic walls.

♦ Porencephaly is usually unilateral and asymmetrical and can be caused by intracranial bleeding.

40 a] Nuchal fold should be measured on the same section as the one for assessing the cerebellum, i.e. suboccipitobregmatic view, by measuring the fat from the outer table of the occiput to the outer border of the skin.

b] NF should normally measure ≤ 6 mm at 18–20 weeks GA. A greater value at this GA may be indicative of Down's syndrome.

41 a] BPD is measured on the transverse section of the fetal skull showing circular skull outline, a short midline echo, cavum septum pellucidum, basal cisterns and thalami. Depending on the chart used, the measurement can be the maximum diameter from the inner border of the skull to the outer border on the opposite side (inner to outer) or from the outer border of the skull to the outer border on the opposite side (outer to outer).

♦ Above section is the BMUS-recommended section for measuring BPD.

♦ In some departments, BPD measurement is taken at the level for assessing the choroid plexus and lateral ventricles.

b] An accurate BPD measurement may be unobtainable due to fetal lie, for example the fetal head may be too deep in the maternal pelvis, or in the direct occipitoanterior (OA) or occipitoposterior (OP) position. Wrong technique can also lead to inaccurate BPD measurement.

c] Problems affecting BPD measurement:
• Fetal problems: spina bifida where the BPD is smaller than expected or ventriculomegaly/hydrocephalus where the BPD is larger than expected.
• Dolichocephaly or brachycephaly: not indicative of fetal problems, merely a variation in the head shape.
• If the measurement is first taken in the 3rd trimester, there is an accuracy variation of up to 2–3 weeks.

— slight rotation of the transducer will demonstrate the femur

— ensure that both ends of the femur are demonstrated.

♦ The femur appears bowed if the medial aspect is demonstrated.

b] Factors in obtaining an inaccurate FL measurement:

— medial femur measured

— humerus measured instead of the femur

— too much gain is used or an abnormal ossification occurs at the distal end of the femur

— only one length is obtained

— faulty callipers.

c] Reduced FL in spite of normal AC and BPD is suggestive of limb deformities. In order to exclude or confirm this diagnosis, check the thoracic cage, ribs and other long bones that are to be measured against the available charts.

97 Fetal face, hands, feet and heart can display subtle ultrasound appearances suggestive of chromosomal abnormality.

98 a] Fetal hands and feet are commonly involved in syndromes of abnormalities. They could be structural markers indicating more serious underlying fetal abnormalities.

b] Chromosomal abnormalities associated with the fetal hands and feet include:

— trisomy 13: polydactyly (i.e. extra digits)

— triploidy: syndactyly (i.e. fused digits)

— trisomy 21: club foot, hypoplasia of 5th finger middle phalanx

— trisomy 18: rockerbottom foot, overlapping fingers and/or clenched fist.

c] Points to note in checking the fetal hands:

— alignment of the hand, fingers and thumb

— number of fingers (any missing or extra digit?)

— ? abnormal thumb position

— ? overlapping fingers

— ? fused digit (syndactyly or ectrodactyly)

— ? small 5th finger due to hypoplasia of the middle phalanx.

d] Points to note in checking the fetal feet:

— alignment and position of the toes

feet angulation, i.e. normal or abnormal (e.g. rockerbottom feet).

♦ In club foot, the sole of the foot and leg will be seen simultaneously with medial deviation on the same plane consistently.

99 • If the diagnosis of a chromosomal abnormality is established before 24/40 then a TOP option can be offered to the patient.

• If the diagnosis is made later in pregnancy then a caesarean section can be avoided for fetal distress during labour.

• Fetal delivery can be planned for, with the attendance of the specialist or at a specialist centre.

• Post-delivery treatment (e.g. surgery) or follow up can be arranged.

• Psychologically and in other ways the couple could prepare for the pregnancy outcome should they want the pregnancy to continue.

100 a] Incidence of trisomy 13 is 1 in 5000. It has a very poor prognosis as less than 5% survive to 3 years of age.

    b] Ultrasound findings suggestive of trisomy 13

Structure	Disorder	Percentage (%)
Head	Holoprosencephaly	75
	Agenesis of corpus callosum	22
	Dandy–Walker syndrome	20
	Hydrocephalus	13
Face	Cleft lip and/or palate	–
	Low set ears	75
Heart	VSD, ASD, PDA	–
	Pulmonary stenosis	80
	Mitral or aortic atresia	–
Abdomen	Omphalocele	30
Kidney	Renal cystic dysplasia	30
	Hydronephrosis	–
Hands and feet	Polydactyly	75

ASD, atrial septal defect; PDA, patent ductus arteriosus; VSD, ventricular septal defect. –, data not available.

101 a] Incidence of trisomy 18 is 1 in 3000; female to male ratio 3:1.

    b] Ultrasound findings suggestive of trisomy 18

Structure	Disorder	Percentage (%)
Hands and feet	Flexed fingers with overlapping fingers	80
	Radial aplasia	–
	Rockerbottom feet	–
Face	Micrognathia	–
	Midline cleft lip and/or palate	–
	Hypotelorism, i.e. close set of eyes with decreased outer to inner ocular distance	–
	Low set 'pixie ears'	15
Head	Hydrocephalus	–
	Agenesis of corpus callosum	–
	Choroid plexus cysts	–
Thorax	Diaphragmatic hernia	–
Heart	VSD, ASD, PDA	–
Abdomen	Omphalocele, oesophageal atresia	–
Kidneys	Cystic dysplasia	–
	Horseshoe kidney	–
Spine	Spina bifida	15
	Growth retardation	100
	Polyhydramnios	–

ASD, atrial septal defect; PDA, patent ductus arteriosus; VSD, ventricular septal defect. –, data not available.

102 a] Incidence of trisomy 21 is 1.3 in 1000.

b] Ultrasound findings suggestive of trisomy 18 include:
— increased nuchal fold
— hypoplasia of 5th finger middle phalanx
— Mild dilatation of renal pelves: > 4 mm at 15–20/40 GA, > 5 mm at 20–30/40 GA, > 7 mm at 30–40/40 GA
— duodenal atresia
— endocardiac cushion defects (atrioventricular canal defects), VSD, ASD, PDA
— cystic hygroma
— hydrops
— omphalocele
— 'sandal gap'.

103 a] Turner's syndrome is the absence of one of the X chromosomes in a female fetus. Incidence is approximately 1 in 5000 live births but it is reported to account for up to 10% of 1st trimester miscarriages.

b] Turner's syndrome is suggested by the ultrasound findings of:
— cystic hygroma
— hydrops
— horseshoe kidney
— hydronephrosis
— renal agenesis
— renal hypoplasia
— cardiac abnormalities (usually coarctation of the aorta).

c] The lethal type of Turner's syndrome presents with nuchal cystic hygroma, generalized oedema, mild pleural effusions, ascites and cardiac abnormalities. The non-lethal type usually does not demonstrate any ultrasound abnormalities.

104 a] Triploidy is caused by the addition of an extra set of chromosomes (three times the haploid chromosome number of 23 = 69 chromosomes).
Triploidy is seen in about 10% of 1st trimester miscarriages.

b] Fetuses with triploidy may exhibit:
— IUGR (early onset) in the 2nd trimester
— oligohydramnios
— hydropic placenta
— cleft lip and/or palate
— micrognathia
— holoprosencephaly, hydrocephalus, agenesis of corpus callosum
— VSD, ASD, PDA
— omphalocele
— hydronephrosis
— renal dysplasia
— fusion of the 3rd and 4th fingers.

♦ 20% of all chromosomal abortuses are thought to be triploid.

♦ Triploidy is invariably lethal. Only a few live births have been described and all have died shortly after birth.

105 a] Fetal hypertelorism is an increased distance between the pupils, or the orbits being too far apart. (Where the distance between the pupils is too short, it is termed fetal hypotelorism.)

b] Hypertelorism can be detected sonographically by measuring the distance between the orbits. In a normal fetus at 20/40, the interobital diameter is similar to ocular diameter, i.e. the distance between the orbits is similar to the width of the orbit itself.

c] Hypertelorism can be caused by:
— hypoplastic greater wings of the sphenoid and overgrowth of the lesser wings of the sphenoid
— a mass lesion such as frontal encephalocele may space the orbits wide apart, thus preventing them reaching their normal anatomical position
— overgrowth of the nasofrontal process of the frontal bone.

d] Hypertelorism can be seen in many syndromes, especially those with cranial contour abnormalities (e.g. those caused by craniosynostosis in fetal alcohol syndrome).

106 a] • SFD or SGA refers to babies born with a birth weight of under 2500 g or under the 10th centile for the GA at which they are delivered. This includes premature babies.
  ♦ Ideally obstetric charts should be derived from the population being studied but in practice standard charts tend to be used.
  ♦ Check the size of the parents and previous siblings (if applicable) and the ethnic group.
 • IUGR is the failure of a fetus to achieve its growth potential. There is no universal definition of IUGR but the criteria may include:
  — very low birth weight (less than 1500 g)
  — low birth weight (less than 2500 g)
  — measuring of relative size – less than the 10th centile, or more than two standard deviations (SD) below the general population mean for the gestational age and sex.
  ♦ The GA of such a fetus must be established before 24/40.
  ♦ Not all IUGR fetuses are SFD or SGA and vice versa.

b] *Intrinsic* factors that influence fetal growth are genetic and endocrine. *Extrinsic* factors include an adequate supply of nutrients from the maternal circulation, efficient maternal–fetal transfer of nutrients, adequate fetal circulation and adequate fetal release of insulin.

c] Accuracy of clinical diagnosis may be poor due to:
— unknown or incorrect menstrual history
— difficulties with obese patients, fibroids or uterine anomalies
— multiple pregnancies – growth rate of one fetus may be impaired.

d] Ultrasound is best for diagnosing IUGR because:
— scans before 20 weeks are accurate for dating pregnancy (BPD will usually predict GA to within ± 5 days)
— the anomaly scan will confirm or refute many structural abnormalities
— follow-up scans can show if the fetal growth pattern is correct

  — serial scans can determine the severity and type of IUGR.
  ♦ 10% of IUGR cases are due to fetal anomaly, thus a careful ultrasound examination of the fetus should be carried out to check for this.

107 'Large for dates' can be the result of:
  — wrong dates
  — multiple pregnancy
  — polyhydramnios
  — macrosomic baby (raises the suspicion of maternal diabetes)
  — coexisting mass with pregnancy (e.g. uterine fibroids or ovarian cysts)
  — end-stage hydrocephaly
  — fetal hydrops.

108 'Small for dates' can be the result of:
  — wrong dates
  — IUD
  — IUGR
  — oligohydramnios
  — SROM
  — genitourinary problems.

109 a] There are three types of IUGR: symmetrical, asymmetrical and femur sparing.
   b] Anatomy of an IUGR fetus should be examined in detail because 10% of IUGR are the result of congenital fetal abnormality. Fetal kidneys and urinary bladder must be examined to exclude renal anomalies.
   c] IUGR is best diagnosed in utero because IUGR fetuses are prone to:
     — increased risk of difficult delivery
     — stunted stature
     — reduced intellect later in life if left untreated in utero.

d] IUGR – causes and problems

Type of IUGR	Description	Causes	Associated problems
Symmetrical	Bonsai babies, i.e. generally small. On the HC:AC graph the ratio will be on or around the mean curve, i.e. head size same as body	Chromosomal anomalies Heroin addiction Ionizing radiation Fetal alcohol syndrome Inadequate maternal nutrition TORCH infections Idiopathic Maternal smoking Genetic factors (e.g. sickle cell disease)	Chromosomal anomaly Intrauterine viral infection Reduced intellect and learning difficulties Short stature Higher incidence of death in the 1st year
Asymmetrical	Long and thin at birth with the appropriate head size for the GA but wasted bodies. On the HC:AC graph, the ratio will be just below or above the mean curve. AC growth slows 2–3 weeks before the HC	Severe maternal cardiac or renal disease Idiopathic (probably due to placental perfusion) Multiple gestation Proteinuric hypertension	Hypoglycaemia Hypothermia Ante- or perinatal asphyxia leading to palsy and/or major mental handicap Neonatal pulmonary haemorrhage Necrotizing enteritis Premature delivery

IUGR – causes and problems – *contd.*

Type of IUGR	Description	Causes	Associated problems
			Hypocalcaemia Stillbirth
Femur sparing	All measurements apart from the femur are small. This type is relatively common. No clinical cause or associated problems have been identified	–	–

TORCH, toxoplasmosis, other infections, rubella, cytomegalovirus, herpes simplex virus.
Other causes of IUGR include placental insufficiency, infectious disease, cardiovascular malformations, teratogens (drugs, chemicals and viruses) and genetic factors.

e] Ultrasound management in symmetrical IUGR:
— detailed ultrasound scan to look for structural abnormalities
— subjective assessment of liquor volume (LV). Reduced LV + symmetrical small for gestational age (SSGA) may indicate renal tract abnormality
— fortnightly ultrasound measurement by the same sonographer and using the same equipment if possible
— Doppler ultrasound measurement.
f] Ultrasound management in asymmetrical IUGR:
— serial ultrasound growth monitoring as above
— LV assessment. Asymmetrical small for gestational age (ASGA) + reduced LV has an increased incidence of perinatal death or handicap
— biophysical profile
— Doppler ultrasound measurement.
g] The ultrasound department should arrange, if possible, the same equipment and the same sonographer for each scan, with a minimum gap between scans of 2 weeks except in very severe cases, in order to reduce errors.
h] Once a month* is usually sufficient for scanning an IUGR fetus but in severe cases this should be done every 2 weeks. This is because weekly scan is prone to more operator error and the growth changes may not be all that significant. (*Depending on the obstetrician and departmental protocol.)

110

Biophysical profile parameter	Score 2	Score 0
Heart rate reactivity	Two or more accelerations in 40 minutes	< 2
Fetal movements	More than three gross body or limb movements in 30 minutes	< 3
Fetal breathing movements (FBM)	At least 30 seconds sustained FBM in 30 minutes	< 30 seconds
Amniotic fluid	More than 1 cm pocket	< 1 cm
Fetal tone	Closed fist or a flexion to extension movement	None

111 In *fetal tone*, fetal extension and flexion movements are closely observed. This could be of the hands or fingers, kicking movements or arching of the spine and its return. *Fetal movement* refers to the gross body or limb movements within the specified time.

112 It is best to assess a growth-retarded fetus approximately 1 hour after maternal feeding as fetal activity is then at its peak.

113 Fetal growth can be assessed using the HC:AC ratio graph. The type of IUGR (if present) can then be confirmed.

114 a] Breech or transverse fetal presentation can be caused by:
— placenta praevia
— cervical fibroid
— ovarian tumour
— fetal abnormalities (e.g. fetal goitre or anencephaly).

b] Fetal weight estimate should be recorded in case of a planned early delivery.

c] Information about the presenting fetal part and the fetal legs, i.e. flexed or extended, should be recorded as this prepares the team for the type of delivery approach.

115 a] Fetal weight estimate is useful in:
— preterm labour
— late 2nd or early 3rd trimester PROM
— multiple pregnancy
— SGA when an early delivery is considered
— non-cephalic presentation
— maternal diabetes mellitus to rule out macrosomia
— an operable fetal condition that is compatible with life but which is deteriorating (e.g. hydronephrosis).

b] Fetal weight can be estimated using AC and HC, and FL and AC. These are preferable to BPD measurement which in late pregnancy may be unreliable due to factors cited in Answer 41g on page 322.

116 Serial ultrasound scans are necessary in women with pregnancy-induced HBP because they commonly have SGA babies. If HBP is complicated by proteinuria, there is an increased risk of placental abruption.

117 Babies born to insulin-dependent mothers are prone to:
— polyhydramnios
— IUGR
— sacral agenesis
— cardiac abnormalities
— macrosomia.

118 Serial ultrasound scans should be performed in pregnant diabetic patients because the fetus is prone to cardiac anomalies and sacral agenesis, for example sirenomelia (mermaid syndrome).
The fetus is also at increased risk of excessive growth (macrosomia) and IUD, and being born as a stillbirth.

- ◆ Diabetic mothers:
  - — carry a risk of having an abnormal baby that is approximately three times that of the normal population
  - — are at an increased risk of pregnancy-induced hypertension, especially pre-eclampsia
  - — are at an increased risk of polyhydramnios, preterm delivery and having an IUGR baby.

119a] Patients referred for anomaly scan

Patient	Factors	Reason
Lady with poorly controlled insulin-dependent diabetes	CNS, heart defects, sacral agenesis (caudal regression syndrome)[a]	These women have a risk that is approximately three times the risk of the normal population in having fetuses with fetal abnormalities
Lady on cocaine[b]	Possible fetal anomalies including CNS anomaly, fetus could be malformed, have limb reductions or missing organs	Maternal exposure may cause fetal vascular disruption or placental vasoconstriction
Lady on warfarin derivatives[c]	1st trimester exposure can result in nasal hypoplasia, chondrodysplasia punctata, IUGR 2nd trimester exposure can result in microcephaly	Can also cause fatal fetal haemorrhage
Lady on lithium[d]	Cardiac anomalies	Possible 10–15% risk of anomalies, especially of the fetal heart because of the teratogenic effect
Lady on diazepam	Cardiac anomalies, spina bifida, cleft lip and/or palate, limb deformity	There are more cardiac defects than in controls
Lady who is a dwarf	FL and long bone measurements and rib cage assessment	To exclude thanatophoric dwarfism of short limbs, narrow chest, protuberant abdomen
Lady on anticonvulsant medication[e]	Face and heart	Exposure of the fetus to antiepileptics introduces a two- to five-fold increased risk of anomalies, especially CHD and oral clefts
Lady who is a chronic alcoholic[f]	CNS anomalies, heart malformations, facial abnormalities, skeletal anomalies, genitourinary malformations Global IUGR and microcephaly may be observed later in the pregnancy	There is an association of chronic maternal alcohol use with fetal congenital defect

[a] Rare abnormality that is seen only in women who suffer from insulin-dependent diabetes. Malformation of the fetus ranges from absent sacrum with short femurs to fused lower limbs (sirenomelia or the mermaid syndrome).
[b] At increased risk of spontaneous abortion, IUGR and premature delivery.
[c] As warfarin could cross the placenta and cause fatal fetal haemorrhage, its use is now contraindicated in pregnancy.
[d] Lithium (used for patients with manic-depressive psychosis) should be considered as a teratogen and should be avoided in pregnancy or in those likely to conceive.
[e] Approximately 1 in 200 pregnant women is epileptic and anticonvulsant therapy is usually continued throughout pregnancy.
[f] Fetus is also prone to IUGR.

♦ In some departments, a diabetic pregnancy, in addition to the regular routine scans, is routinely scanned for growth and liquor volume at 28, 32 and 36 weeks (Doppler is indicated if < 3rd centile).

b] Patients referred for growth scan

Patient	Factors	Reason
Lady who suffers from SLE[a]	IUGR	Antibodies and anticoagulants can cross placenta and cause macrocoagulation at the placenta bed
Lady who suffers from uncontrolled sickle cell disease	IUGR	Due to chronic hypoxia and anaemia
Lady who is a heavy cigarette smoker (≥ 20 a day)	IUGR	See Answer 130 (p. 350)
Lady who is known HIV positive[b]	IUGR	Especially if mother is badly affected
Lady with pre-eclampsia	IUGR	Tends to mirror the same mechanism as SLE at placenta level
Lady with poorly controlled insulin-dependent diabetes	Macrosomia, polyhydramnios; a small minority will have microsomic or IUGR fetus	Maternal hyperglycaemia will cause fetal hyperglycaemia which stimulates fetal hyperinsulinaemia
Lady on cocaine	IUGR	Cocaine is known to be appetite suppressing, raising the possibility of nutritional deficiency

[a] Patients with SLE are said to have high fetal losses.
[b] It is unclear if this could cause fetal CNS problems.
Please refer to the textbooks in the Further reading section for a comprehensive list.

♦ In some departments, routinely, pregnant women with:
— sickle cell disease are scanned for growth and liquor volume at 28, 32 and 36 weeks (Doppler is done if fetal growth is < 3rd centile)
— lupus are scanned for growth, liquor volume and Doppler twice weekly (fortnightly) from 24 weeks.
— hypertension are scanned for growth, liquor volume and Doppler at 28, 32 and 36 weeks
— diabetes are scanned for growth, liquor volume at 28, 32 and 36 weeks (Doppler is done if fetal growth is < 3rd centile.)

120 a] Congenital abnormality is more prevalent in monozygotic twins.
   b] Multiple pregnancy should be scanned in line with deparmental protocol (growth charts must be plotted and preferably with a diagram of fetal positions).
   ♦ In some departments in addition to the two routine scans offered to most women in pregnancy:
   — monochorionic twins are also scanned at 16 weeks and for growth and liquor volumes twice weekly (fortnightly) from 24 weeks
   — dichorionic twins are scanned for growth and liquor volumes at 28, 32 and 36 weeks.

— high-risk pregnancies are best scanned on the day of the ANC appointment but shortly before the appointment if possible. This has many advantages including the fact that the obstetricians will be more available if needed, the scan findings will be most current and it saves the patient an extra hospital visit for scanning.

c] Multiple pregnancy is prone to:
— twin–twin transfusion syndrome (seen in monozygotic twins)
— disparity in size and growth
— acardiac acephalic monster
— stuck twin
— vanishing twin
— death of a twin
— IUD of both twins, especially if they are monozygotic.

d] TTTS is a condition in which blood is shunted from one twin to the other. It causes minimal impairment of growth in its least severe state. In its most severe state it produces anaemia, hydrops fetalis in the smaller twin and polycythaemia in the other twin. Polyhydramnios is common.
◆ To treat this condition, endoscopic laser photocoagulation of the abnormal vessels may be performed at a specialized Fetal Medicine Unit.

e] The body components of conjoined twins can be seen on ultrasound to move together. They are partially fused and they are always MC/MA. Polyhydramnios is common.
◆ Conjoined twins are due to an incomplete anatomical separation at some location in MZ twins. Incidence is quoted as approximately 1:50 000 to 1:100 000 births.
◆ The sonographer must note the number of heads, hearts, trunks and limbs in the scan report.

f] Survival of conjoined twins is dependent on GA at delivery, the type and extent of the union between the twins, and the presence of associated organ malformation.

The four main types of conjoined twins

Type of twin	Description	Percentage of conjoined twins (%)
Thoracopagus	Joined at the sternum, diaphragm and liver	75
Pygopagus	Joined both at the lower back and sacrum	18
Ischiopagus	Connected from umbilicus to a fused pelvis and having three or four legs	5
Cranopagus	Fused at the skull. They have separate brains but frequently a common venous drainage	2

g] Stuck twin syndrome is a fetal condition in which there is severe oligohydramnios around one twin and polyhydramnios around the second twin. The stuck twin will not move when the mother's position is changed and may appear to be adhered to the anterior or lateral aspect of the uterus. Magnified view will show the membrane alongside the fetus and this twin is usually much the smaller of the two. This syndrome is mostly related to the twin–twin transfusion syndrome and often only one placenta is seen. This usually develops about 22/40 but may be seen earlier.

◆ Repeated amniotic fluid drainage from the twin with polyhydramnios is said to increase the chance of the twins' survival. Such twins will require more frequent ultrasound assessment as decided by the obstetrician.

◆ Structural abnormalities that may imply chromosomal problems should be excluded.

121 An acardiac acephalic monster is an unusual variant of a MZ/MC twin or triplet pregnancy. A twin is seen with no heart or head but may show movement. This twin will show massive skin thickening and other structural abnormalities including omphalocele and two-vessel cord. Reversed blood flow to the abdomen using colour-flow Doppler may be noted. Either no membrane or a thin membrane is seen. Polyhydramnios is seen around the normal twin and severe oligohydramnios around the acardiac twin.

◆ Check whether the normal twin shows signs of fetal hydrops.

◆ Care must be taken that the acardiac twin is not mistaken as an anencephalic twin with no FHB.

◆ In specialist FMUs, laser ablation may be done so that the normal twin will have a better chance of survival.

122 Fetal risks associated with multiple gestation include:
— congenital abnormality
— TTTS
— stuck twin syndrome
— death of a co-twin (see Answer 84 in Ch. 4, p. 287)
— IUGR
— preterm labour or delivery
— technical difficulties at delivery
— cord prolapse
— birth asphyxia
— higher risk of cot death.

123 Maternal risks associated with multiple gestation include:
— anaemia
— antepartum haemorrhage
— nausea and vomiting of early pregnancy
— miscarriage and the 'vanishing twin' syndrome
— increased minor disorders of pregnancy
— hypertension and pre-eclampsia
— polyhydramnios
— gestational diabetes
— increased risk of operative delivery and caesarean section
— PPH.

124 Major congenital abnormalities in MZ twins include:
— conjoined twins, quoted as occurring at a rate of 0.5%
— acardiac twins, quoted as occurring at a rate of 1%
— congenital heart disease
— bowel atresia.

125 Conditions that may affect twins in utero include:
   — polyhydramnios
   — death of one twin
   — IUGR.
   ◆ Polyhydramnios:
      — may occur in one gestational sac, typically in TTTS or 'stuck twin'. The
        perinatal mortality rate is quoted as > 80%
      — may be in association with congenital abnormality or gestational diabetes
      — cause may not be known in an acute case in MZ twins.

126 In twin pregnancy polyhydramnios can cause:
   — preterm labour
   — rupture of membrane
   — placental abruption
   — malpresentation
   — cord accidents.

127 Incidence of death of one twin is quoted as 6% in association with TTTS or in
   isolation.
   ◆ The risk of death for the surviving twin is quoted as 20% due to premature
     delivery; it is higher in MZ twins.

128 Serial ultrasound scans are recommended because of the risk of:
   — poor growth in one or both fetus(es) and therefore to identify IUGR or detect
     growth discordance
   — polyhydramnios
   — preterm delivery
   — placenta praevia
   and also to identify TTTS.

129 a] Ultrasound findings that confirm IUD include:
      — lack of fetal heartbeats
      — lack of fetal movement
      — depending on the time of death and scan:
         • discrepancy between GA and fetus size
         • overlapping skull bones
         • skin and/or scalp oedema (subcutaneous oedema), seen as a double
           outline surrounding the fetus
      — unnatural extreme flexion or extension
      — loss of definition of features in the fetal trunk; there may be echoes within
        the fetal brain
      — gas in the fetal abdomen which may make fetal anatomy assessment
        difficult if not impossible
      — maceration causes echoes to develop in the amniotic fluid.
      ◆ It is best that IUD be confirmed by two qualified sonographers and
        documented in the report.
      ◆ Subcutaneous oedema is also seen in fetal hydrops and fetuses of patients
        with maternal diabetes.
   b] Causes of IUD include:
      — unrectified factors causing fetal distress

137 • Larger chamber(s) are caused by the chamber(s) receiving more blood flow than normal which may be due to diversion flow from the other side of the heart or due to valve regurgitation or obstructed valve.
  • Smaller chamber(s) are caused by the chamber(s) receiving less blood flow than normal.

138 • RV – severe pulmonary incompetence; severe pulmonary stenosis (rare)
  • RA – tricuspid regurgitation; Ebstein's anomaly
  • LV – severe aortic stenosis; severe aortic incompetence (rare)
  • LA – mitral regurgitation.

139 • RV – tricuspid atresia; pulmonary atresia with intact septum
  • LV – mitral atresia; mitral and aortic atresia (hypoplastic left heart).

140 • Small PA – hypoplastic right heart; Ebstein's anomaly with pulmonary hypoplasia
  • Small aorta – coarctation; hypoplastic left heart
  • Large aorta – tetralogy of Fallot; truncus arteriosus.

141 a] Fetal tachycardia is when the fetal heart beats very fast, with a quoted rate of over 200 beats per minute (bpm).
  b] Fetal tachycardia is considered pathological and may require treatment whether the tachycardia is intermittent or sustained.

142 Fetal brachycardia is when the fetal heartbeat is slow, rate quoted as under 100 bpm.

143 Irregular heart rhythm in fetuses 30 weeks or more GA is a common finding and structural abnormality should be excluded.
  ◆ Irregular heart rhythm is considered to be benign in the absence of any structural abnormality.

144 Referral to a specialized fetal cardiologist will depend on the departmental protocol but has been advised in cases of:
  — cardiac abnormality
  — irregular rhythm in the presence of structural abnormality
  — tachycardia whether sustained or intermittent
  — sustained bradycardia.

145 The LVOT demonstrates the LV and aortic outflow tract. The anterior wall of the aorta is seen in continuity with the interventricular septum without any step or break. The aorta is also seen as having a sweeping course towards the fetal right shoulder.
  ◆ The mitral valve is seen but not the tricuspid valve.
  ◆ A break may indicate the presence of a ventricular septal defect.

146 The RVOT demonstrates the PA leaving the RV and pointing backwards towards the fetal spine with continuity with the arterial duct.

147 The transverse arches plane demonstrates:
  — PA in continuity with the duct (it is also the more anterior vessel)
  — aortic arch
  — superior vena cava.

- The width of the aortic arch and pulmonary artery/ductal arch should be approximately equal in width at about 20/40 GA, as later in the pregnancy the PA tends to be slightly larger than the Ao.

148 Assessment of the ventricular septum is important so that ventricular septal defect (VSD) can be excluded. VSDs have associations with extracardiac anomalies.

149 a] An AVSD is when the atrial septum does not meet the crux.
- AVSD is associated with a high incidence of chromosomal abnormalities and is a component of more complex heart defects.
- A careful examination of the crux will help in diagnosing AVSD.

b] A VSD can involve malalignment of components of the septum plus a hole; it may also be a hole in the ventricular septum of a normal heart.
- A careful examination of the LVOT will help in diagnosing VSD.

150 A true pericardial effusion should extend across the atrioventricular junction, be at least 2 mm in width and visible on multiple heart planes.

151 For confirmed pericardial effusion, karyotyping and screening for infection is indicated. Tapping of the effusion may be indicated should there be tamponade.

152 Causes of pericardial effusion include:
— unknown aetiology in a small effusion is not uncommon
— anaemia
— cardiac dysfunction from any other cause
— chromosomal abnormalities
— congenital infection
— severe placental insufficiency
— structural heart defects.

153 a] Fig. 5.153a, abdominal situs; Fig. 5.153b, 4-chamber view; Fig. 5.153c, LVOT.

b] **A5.153b**

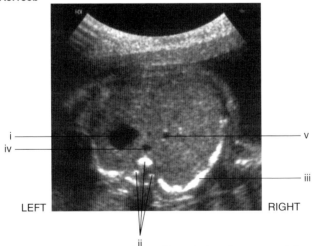

Labelling in Fig. A5.153b is confirmed since in a normal fetus the fetal stomach is on the left.

Obstetrics – 2nd and 3rd trimester, part two

ANSWERS

1 a] Fig. 6.1 shows a transverse section demonstrating the lateral ventricles. This section is cephalad to the section for measuring the recommended BMUS biparietal diameter (BPD).

b] Ultrasound shows an increased anterior ventricular hemisphere ratio (AVHR) and posterior ventricular hemisphere ratio (PVHR) of 15/22, 15/22 (normal value is ≤ 0.5). Head circumference (HC) is not enlarged.

c] Differential diagnosis is ventriculomegaly and hydrocephalus, seen in communicating hydrocephalus, severe ventriculomegaly, normal variant and aqueduct stenosis.

d] The fetal liver should also be checked for calcifications and signs of hydrops.

e] Karyotyping and screen infection were performed to exclude the possible cause of these ultrasound findings. Causes include trisomy 18, 13 or 21, fetal infection and translocations 7p and 9p.

f] Ultrasound can be used in future management to assess fetal growth scans and well-being of this fetus and to monitor any change in fetal head size and anatomy.

♦ Some authors suggest that:
— mild lateral ventricular dilatation could be 10–15 mm
— ventriculomegaly is diagnosed when the atrium is ≥ 11 mm at any GA and that it is associated with central nervous system (CNS) abnormality.

♦ Before 24/40 in cases of associated spina bifida, the HC may be small rather than large.

2 a] Structure a = eye socket; b = nose; c = upper lip. There is a gap in the lip on the right which extends up to the nose and into the palate. This is a unilateral right cleft lip and palate.

b] Incidence is approximately 1 in 700 to 1 in 1000 live births.

c] Cleft lip and/or palate is caused by failure of the lip to fuse by day 35 which may impair palate shelf closure at 8–9 weeks GA. This has been attributed to genetic and environmental factors such as multifactional inheritance and chromosomal abnormalities (e.g. trisomy 13 or single-gene trait); it may be isolated, or associated with maternal drug treatment, especially anticonvulsants.

d] Ultrasound may be used in:
— exclusion of any other structural abnormality
— ultrasound-guided amniocentesis to exclude chromosomal abnormalities

— routine growth scans to assess fetal growth

— assessing the amniotic fluid volume as the fetus is at risk of polyhydramnios due to swallowing defects.

It is important that amniotic band, congenital heart disease (CHD) and intracranial abnormalities are excluded.

3 a] Ultrasound is of a transverse section of the fetal head demonstrating the short midline, the thalami and the cavum septum pellucidum.

b] The fetal cranium appears intact but posterior to the occiput is a multiple cystic structure with thin septa within it.

c] Diagnosis is most probably cystic hygroma with the differentials being encephalocele or meningocele.

d] Associated findings include Turner's syndrome (45 XO) or trisomy 21, 18 or 13, or other syndromes that are similar to Turner's or trisomy 18. It may be associated with hydronephrosis, renal hypoplasia, renal agenesis and generalized hydrops.

Amniocentesis will help confirm the fetal genotype. An ultrasound search should be conducted for any associated structural abnormalities usually seen in Turner's syndrome or trisomy 21, 18 and 13 fetuses, such as heart defects and ultrasound findings suggestive of hydrops and renal problems.

e] Cervical lymphatic vessel obstruction may be the cause of the problem in this fetus.

4 a] Ultrasound appearance is of a 9 mm hyperechoic linear structure posterior to the lower lumbosacral spine. The overlying skin covering is intact.

b] Diagnosis is spina bifida occulta.

c] Spina bifida occulta occurs in L5 or S1 vertebrae in about 10% of otherwise normal people. It usually does not produce any clinical symptoms, but a small percentage of affected infants have significant functional defects of the underlying spinal cord and spinal roots.

♦ Spina bifida can be associated with chromosomal abnormality (e.g. triploidy, trisomy 13 and 18), obesity, use of antiepileptic drugs (e.g. sodium valproate) and maternal overheating in the 1st trimester.

♦ Women with diabetes have a high risk of neural tube defect (NTD) of 2% but this is more likely to be anencephaly than spina bifida.

5 a] The sonographer should be concerned about Lady A's fetus as no normal 4C view of the heart was obtained. The same concern applies to Lady B as no normal left ventricle is demonstrated.

b] Both ladies would benefit from specialist echocardiography to ascertain what may be wrong with the fetal hearts and the possible outcome. Other structural abnormalities should be excluded.

♦ Lady A's fetus was later confirmed to be CHD situs solitus with a ventricular septal defect (VSD). Lady B's fetus was later confirmed to have a hypoplastic left ventricle.

♦ In both fetuses no other structural abnormality was seen.

6 a] Ultrasound shows the stomach bubble and urinary bladder; another cystic area is demonstrated in the fetal abdomen.

16 a] • Find out if there is any history of chromosomal abnormality on her side, i.e. siblings or immediate family members.
Why:
— Any family history on the lady's side will increase the chances of this pregnancy having a chromosomal abnormality.

• From the notes or asking the patient, the sonographer needs to establish what follow-up test was offered to the patient following her NT screening scan and what her response to this was, e.g. was CVS or another invasive technique suggested and what was her reponse to this?
Why:
— At the age of 42 years, she is classified as in the 'high risk group'.
— According to the maternal adjusted risk of 1:230, she is equally classified as being in the 'high risk group' although the 1:230 result is a lot better than her initial age-related risk of 1:38, the cut off being 1:250 or 1:300 in hospitals that run the 1st trimester ultrasound screening programme.
— Being a primid at age 42, this is most likely to be a 'precious pregnancy'.
— Bilateral renal pelvis dilatation and choroid plexus cysts are two 'soft markers', irrespective of the patient's age, for which normally patients are counselled to consider an invasive test such as amniocentesis in order to check the chromosomal status of the fetus.
— These findings will normally further increase the risk of a chromosomal problem in the fetus.
— If lady Z had a CVS or amniocentesis and the chromosomal result was normal then further scans to monitor CPC and kidneys will have to be organised in line with departmental protocol.
— If on the other hand, invasive testing was offered but declined initially, this result will further make the need for one more advisable.
— Depending on departmental protocol, this lady may have to be referred for a specialist fetal cardiac scan.

b] These ultrasound findings will affect the previously given maternal adjusted risk of lady Z.
How:
— Each soft marker will increase the risk of chromosomal abnormality in this fetus. With two soft markers, the risk will be significantly increased.

c] the sonographer should try to exclude or confirm any of the following:
— increased nuchal fold
— echogenic foci in the fetal heart
— echogenic bowels
— sandal gap
— rock bottom foot
— clinodactyly
— short femur
— clasped or overlapping fingers
— single umbilical artery.
Why:
— To exclude or confirm structural abnormalities that are known to be peculiar to chromosomal abnormalities such as trisomy 18 or 21.

◆ CPC is mostly associated with trisomy 18 and possibly trisomy 21.

d] — Should the lady opt for invasive testing, it would be under ultrasound control.

— Specialist heart scans if this has not be done previously.

— Follow-up scans to monitor fetal growth plus assess the fetal kidneys and CPC.

e] — This result needs to be communicated sensitively and carefully.

— Lady Z will need a referral for her to be seen by the obstetrician or/and agreed FMU as soon as possible.

◆ In some departments, high-risk pregnancies following NT screening scan are classified as:

a. woman who are 35 years old and above

b. irrespective of maternal age, women whose maternal adjusted risk following NT measurement is less than 1 in 250, e.g. as 1 in 230 in this case

c. women who qualify to be in groups a and b above at the same time like lady Z.

◆ These ladies/couples are counselled following their 1st trimester NT screening scan with regard to considering further testing. Those who decline further tests are given the following three options to choose from:

1. talk to the screening midwife before leaving the ANC

2. given relevant information leaflets to take home to read and contact the ANC at a later date should they change their minds regarding invasive testing

3. refuse further information and further testing.

◆ Whatever the lady/couple's choice is, it is documented in her hospital records.

17 a] Ultrasound shows a single fetus. FHB and movements were reported as seen. Fetal measurements are equal to dates. Some fluid is shown above and to the left of the posterior placenta and inferior to the amnion. Depth of one of the pockets of free fluid measured is 3.86 cm. This is most probably a detached amnion.

b] Causes of leaking liquor:

— SROM

— following invasive examination such as amniocentesis or chorionic villi sampling (CVS)

— following severe direct trauma to the maternal abdomen

— as a sign of early premature labour.

c] In the long term SROM may cause:

— oligohydramnios

— deviated hands and club feet

— pulmonary hypoplasia

— premature labour and delivery

— IUD.

d] • Present management: check FHB, check fetal growth and well-being, find any ultrasound evidence for the leakage, assess liquor volume, assess the length of the cervix and maternal internal os to exclude cervical incompetence, assess fetal renal anatomy.

• Future management: as above and to monitor the liquor volume. This may include twice weekly biophysical profiles and fortnightly scans.

◆ Finding a short cervical length with some fluid in the internal os is suggestive of premature rupture of the membranes (PROM).

42 a] Straightened, lying alongside each other, are the lower limbs (? complete fusion) which were reported as moving together.

   b] This is most likely to be sirenomelia (mermaid syndrome).

   c] Patients with insulin-dependent diabetes mellitus are more susceptible to having a sirenomelic fetus.

   ◆ Sirenomelia was later confirmed.

43 a] Structure a = testis; b = hydrocele; c = femur.

   b] Bilateral hydrocele is demonstrated in this male fetus. This may be due to intra-abdominal pathology such as ascites or an intra-abdominal cyst and sometimes no pathology is identified.

   c] The presence or absence of ascites or intra-abdominal pathology should be checked (see Answer 76 in Ch. 5, p. 330).

   ◆ Where no intra-abdominal pathology is found, hydroceles tend to resolve postnatally or can be corrected surgically.

      ◆ No other structural abnormality was seen in this fetus.

44 a] Structure a = right foot; b = right knee; c = fetal abdomen; d = left foot; e = left knee; f = left fibula.

   b] On ultrasound the right leg is shorter than the left leg as seen in Fig. 6.44a. The right foot appears abnormal as seen in Fig. 6.44b. The left fibula as shown in Fig. 6.44c is 27 mm whilst the right fibula is approximately 19 mm.

   c] Ultrasound should be used to:
   — assess other limbs
   — exclude other structural abnormality
   — subsequently monitor fetal growth and well-being (should the parents wish to continue with the pregnancy).

   ◆ Whether or not any ultrasound-guided invasive testing is done will depend on the clinician and the parents as this finding could indicate the rare possibility of a genetic syndrome.

   ◆ Ultrasound findings were confirmed and no other structural abnormality was identified. At postmortem a vestigial right foot was found.

45 a] Structure i = spine; ii = mass; iii = membrane. Fig. 6.45a and b, sagittal views of the fetal abdomen; Fig. 6.45c and d, transverse views of the fetal abdomen.

   b] Ultrasound showed a defect in the abdominal wall with a protruding mass surrounded by some fluid and covered by a membrane.

   c] This probably represents an omphalocele. The differential diagnosis is umbilical hernia.

   Clinical significance: 25–50% of fetuses with omphalocele have an associated chromosomal abnormality, especially trisomy 13 and 18, or cardiac lesions. A search for other soft markers and a detailed cardiac scan are important.

   ◆ MSAFP screening is quoted as being able to detect up to 40% of omphaloceles.

   ◆ Karyotyping the fetus will confirm its chromosomal status.

   ◆ See Answers 121 in Chapter 4 (p. 296) and 55 in Chapter 5 (p. 326).

   ◆ Omphalocele was later confirmed.

46 a] Ultrasound showed a thick membrane extending from the anterior to the posterior wall, giving the appearance of dividing the gestational sac into two parts.

b] This probably represents an amniotic sheet. Differential diagnosis includes twin gestational sac membrane but in such a case, the remains from the blighted ovum will enclose a small space. It is unlikely to be amniotic bands as these are thinner and less pronounced.

c] The sonographer should also note in the report if any fetal part (e.g. a limb) is caught in or by this structure.

d] The pregnancy will be unaffected as there is no pathological significance associated with amniotic sheet.

- Amniotic sheet is due to a gestational sac implanting on the membrane of a previously existing synechia in the uterus before conception. The amnion and chorion around the synechia give it the double layer. Amniotic membrane is thinner than amniotic sheet.
- The same appearance was noted earlier in this singleton pregnancy at the 1st trimester scan. No fetal part was noted to be caught in or by this structure.

47 a] On ultrasound the left renal pelvis is dilated, AP diameter being 5 mm; the right renal pelvis AP diameter was 9 mm. The urinary bladder is demonstrated with no obvious overdistension.

b] Renal pelvis dilatation may be suggestive of renal problems in this fetus or be a soft marker for trisomy 21. It is important that other structural abnormalities be confirmed or excluded and the fetal sex ascertained. (The parents' wish to be told or not be told the fetal sex could still be respected.) It is helpful to ask the couple if there is any family history of renal problems.

c] Future ultrasound management:

— in the absence of any other soft marker, perform a growth scan to monitor fetal growth and well-being and to assess any changes in the fetal kidneys

— in the presence of any other marker, ultrasound-guided invasive testing may be indicated depending on departmental protocol and the parents' wish.

— arrange postnatal follow-up scans if clinically indicated.

- Fetus was male.
- Father had a nephrostomy when he was under 3 years of age and another relative had renal problems.
- The above findings were confirmed. No other structural abnormality was found.

48 a] See Charts 13, 14, 15, 16 (pp 427–430 in the Appendix).

b] At 23/40 fetal AC is on the 3rd centile. BPD and HC are on the 10th centile and FL is below the 3rd centile for GA. One would expect a normal or longer FL due to the quoted parental height. The fact that the fetal measurements are on the 10th centile or below it should raise concern as to the well-being of this fetus.

Depending on the departmental protocol:

— structural abnormalities need to be excluded again

— uterine and umbilical artery Dopplers should be carried out or suggested to the referring clinician. There may be a need for middle cerebral artery (MCA) Doppler

— serial growth scans should be performed to confirm or exclude IUGR and type, late onset of any structural abnormality, and to monitor amniotic fluid volume.

- Chromosomal or syndromic problems may need to be excluded.

displacement to the right although the apical orientation of the heart is unaffected. No obvious polyhydramnios or placentomegaly is demonstrated or indicated. Differential diagnoses include cystic adenomatoid malformation (CAM), diaphragmatic hernia, bronchogenic or enteric cyst and lung sequestration.

b] The sonographer should note the presence or absence of any other structural abnormality (CAM has no relationship with chromosomal abnormality whereas diaphragmatic hernia is often associated with trisomy 18 and 21). Fetal hydrops, polyhydramnios and placentomegaly, which are common features of CAM, need to be excluded.

c] Follow-up scans will be required for this fetus to exclude any chromosomal abnormality, establish the diagnosis, assess fetal growth and well-being and monitor the ultrasound findings.

55 a] Ultrasound shows that there are six toes instead of the normal five; this is characteristic of polydactyly.

b] This could be an isolated finding but may also be seen as part of a chromosomal abnormality including trisomy 13, 18 and 21 or be part of one of the abnormalities seen in many syndromes.

56 a] Ultrasound shows small hypoechoic/cystic areas within a hyperechoic area in the left thoracic region (measurements not included). There appears to be cardiac displacement to the right although apical orientation of the heart is unaffected.

b] Differential diagnoses include CAM, bronchogenic or enteric cyst, lung sequestration and diaphragmatic hernia.

57 a] On ultrasound there is little brain tissue above the level of the fetal eyes and the cranium is absent – possible artefact or abnormality of one of the orbits.

b] Differential diagnosis is anencephaly or iniencephaly.

c] Crown–rump length (CRL) in most cases will be less than expected for GA. BPD and HC will be unobtainable due to the lack of the cranium. This fetus can be dated by using femur length instead.

d] This is invariably a lethal condition.

58 a] Ultrasound shows fluid in the cervical canal, possibly representing herniation of the amniotic sac without fetal parts, and an internal os width of 3.3 cm. Cervical length was not included but appears almost non-existent.

b] This most likely represents an incompetent cervix in the 2nd trimester.

c] This pregnancy is susceptible to miscarriage or preterm delivery.

d] Further ultrasound assessment using a TVS with an empty maternal urinary bladder (if not contraindicated and depending on the patient's wish) may be useful.

◆ See Answer 4 in Chapter 5 (pp 306–307).

59 a] Ultrasound shows blunting of the sinciput (lemon sign) and a banana-shaped cerebellum (Arnold–Chiari malformation).

b] Both findings are suggestive of a coexisting spina bifida.

60 a] Ultrasound shows multiple echogenic foci within the liver capsule.

b] Ultrasound can be used to exclude any other structural defect and in ultrasound-guided testing to confirm the chromosomal status of the fetus.

◆ Hepatic calcification may be single or multiple ≤ 2 mm in diameter echogenic foci within the liver capsule or liver substance. This may be isolated and of no pathological significance but may be seen in association with chromosomal abnormality or congenital infections.

◆ Perihepatic calcification was later confirmed.

61 a] Ultrasound shows an arachnoid septa traversing the CM.

b] This is a normal finding with no clinical significance.

62 a] Structure i = nose; ii = upper lip; iii = lower lip; iv = chin.

b] Ultrasound shows coronal view of the chin, lips and nose.

c] On ultrasound there is an echo-free gap in the upper lip.

d] This is most likely a unilateral cleft lip and/or palate.

e] Cleft lip and/or palate may be an isolated finding, may be multifactorial or can be associated with chromosomal abnormalities, including triploidy, trisomy 18 or 21, or certain syndromes, or may be seen in fetuses of women on medication including diazepam, steroids, phenytoin and carbamazepine, or seen with the use of alcohol.

◆ Careful assessment of the fetus – especially the brain and heart to exclude other structural abnormalities – is important.

◆ Central cleft lip and/or palate is usually associated with other brain abnormalities and facial problems, including proboscis, hypotelorism and trisomy 13.

◆ The amniotic fluid may be increased where there are problems with fetal swallowing but otherwise it will be normal.

◆ Cleft lip and/or palate may be unilateral, bilateral, on either side or in the midline.

◆ Chromosomal abnormality is found postnatally in < 1% of babies with facial cleft.

63 a] See Answer 51d above.

b] The waveforms show bilateral notches in the uterine arteries; the PI on each side is 2.63. There is reversed end diastolic flow in the umbilical artery.

◆ Abnormal waveforms in the umbilical arteries have been reported as an early sign of fetal impairment.

◆ It has been suggested that pre-eclampsia and IUGR are associated with an inadequate quality and quantity of the maternal vascular response to placentation.

◆ Reversed end diastolic frequency (EDF) in the umbilical artery is associated with a high perinatal mortality and increased incidence of lethal structural and chromosomal defects in the fetus.

c] Future ultrasound management should include serial monitoring of fetal growth and well-being, and amniotic fluid and Doppler studies, including the MCA.

64 a] Ultrasound shows a dilated upper pole of the kidney and a crescent-shaped line in the urinary bladder.

b] Duplex collecting system is the most likely diagnosis.

c] This finding can affect the urinary bladder as a ureterocele is an associated finding. A large urinary bladder is seen where the ureterocele disrupts fetal urination.

d] The sonographer should confirm the sex of the fetus. Ureteroceles are more often seen in females; vesicoureteric junction obstruction is more common in males.

e] Ultrasound can be useful in detailed echocardiography, ultrasound-guided invasive testing and serial monitoring of fetal well-being.

◆ Duplex collecting system in the absence of hydronephrosis may be difficult to diagnose in utero.

b] Ultrasound shows an increased nuchal fold and plural effusion; a cardiac defect cannot be excluded.

c] Future ultrasound management should include a detailed heart scan to rule out any cardiac defect. Other structural abnormality would need to be excluded. Serial ultrasound scans will be useful in assessing fetal growth and well-being.

84 a] In deciding how to describe the kidney in Fig. 6.84a, the sonographer should compare the echogenicity of the kidney with that of the fetal lungs.

b] On ultrasound the kidney appears echogenic (the measurement is not included so it is difficult to comment on its size in relation to fetal GA). The urinary bladder is grossly distended and posterior to it is a possible dilated urethra, 'keyhole' sign or posterior urethral valve.

♦ Microcysts within a kidney will make that kidney appear more echogenic than the fetal lungs.

c] The scan report should include:
— the amniotic fluid assessment
— evidence of any other ultrasound-identifiable structural abnormality
— the fetal sex.

♦ Posterior urethral valve is seen only in the male fetus, with reduced or no amniotic fluid.

♦ Should this urinary bladder appearance be seen in a female fetus megacystic microcolon syndrome should be suspected. This is often accompanied by polyhydramnios.

d] Echogenic kidneys or microscopic kidneys are suggestive of infantile polycystic kidney disease which usually affects both fetal kidneys. This disease is described as lethal with the possibility of a 1 in 4 chance of recurrence (autosomal recessive inheritance pattern). It is estimated that 1 in 5 fetuses with posterior urethral valves will have a chromosomal abnormality, especially trisomy 21, 18 and 13.

e] Future ultrasound management may include:
— a detailed scan, including cardiac scan, to rule out any other structural abnormality
— draining the urinary bladder under ultrasound control (depending on departmental protocol and the parents' wish)
— ultrasound-guided invasive testing to establish the chromosomal status of the fetus
— performing serial ultrasound scans to assess fetal kidney size as there is a tendency for their growth (if it is microscopic kidneys) throughout the pregnancy, and to monitor fetal growth and well-being.

85 a] Ultrasound shows this fetal upper limb to be flexed and immobile.

b] Distal arthrogryposis is the most likely diagnosis.

♦ Other peripheral joints such as the fetal feet and jaw may be affected.

♦ It is important to search for any soft markers which may indicate that this finding is part of a genetic syndrome.

c] The sonographer should also check the amniotic fluid volume and for the presence or absence of fetal hydrops because both features are usually seen alongside fixed, immobile limbs in bizarre positions in fetuses with multiple congenital contractures (arthrogryposis multiplex congenita).

♦ Uterine anomalies and fibroids within the uterus which may cause constriction also need to be excluded.

d] Distal arthrogryposis is described as being autosomal dominant and arthrogryposis multiplex congenita as being autosomal recessive.

♦ This was later confirmed to be distal arthrogryposis.

86 a] Ultrasound shows a defect in the skull (measurement not indicated) through which some brain tissue has herniated.

b] Encephalocele is the most likely diagnosis. Differential diagnosis is cystic hygroma but in this there will be no defect in the fetal skull.

c] The HC will be small and is most likely to be below the 5th centile for GA due to the herniated brain tissue outside the fetal skull.

d] Ultrasound will detect this lesion because encephalocele has a skin covering (in some cases there may be leakage of CSF).

e] Encephalocele may be associated with some syndromes and chromosomal abnormalities, brain or cardiac abnormalities, facial clefts and genital malformation.

f]

Diagnostic test	Reason
Ultrasound-guided invasive test	To confirm or exclude chromosomal abnormality
MRI or CT	To assess the defect and confirm or exclude CNS abnormality
Detailed echocardiography	To rule out any cardiac defect

♦ Normal ossification of the vault is complete by 12/40.

♦ Amniotic band syndrome should be excluded as this could be a a reason for this finding.

87 a] Ultrasound shows a cystic structure in the posterior horn of the lateral ventricle of the fetal brain (measurements not included).

b] Differential diagnoses include porencephalic cyst, arachnoid cyst, intracranial bleed and vein of Galen aneurysm.

c] This entity can be confirmed by:
— obtaining ventricular measurements using the AVHR and PVHR to rule out ventriculomegaly or obstructive hydrocephaly
— using colour-flow Doppler: flow will be seen if this structure is a vein of Galen aneurysm but no flow if it is an arachnoid cyst.

d] The sonographer should also record the presence or absence of any other structural abnormality which might be suggestive of a chromosomal abnormality, especially trisomy 18.

e] Ultrasound can be useful to assess fetal growth and well-being and to monitor the fetal head (especially AVHR and PVHR) and cyst size.

    — patients at high risk including:
- where there is a family history of first-degree relatives with CHD
- mothers who suffer from collagen vascular disease, diabetes, phenylketonuria or CHD
- mothers who have been exposed to a teratogen such as valproic acid, lithium carbonate, phenytoin, alcohol or isotretinoin, anti-convulsants
- patients on drugs
- patients who have been exposed to rubella or infected by mumps, CMV, toxoplasmosis or coxsackie virus

    — anatomical extracardiac abnormality such as diaphragmatic hernia or severe polyhydramnios, or in a chromosomal abnormality

    — abnormal fetal heart rate

    — non-immune hydrops fetalis.

c] • Transposition of the great arteries: this is suggested by parallel great arteries instead of the aortic/pulmonary arteries crossing over at approximately right angles near their origins. Complete transposition is one of the most difficult cardiac lesions to recognize in utero. In most cases, the 4C view is normal, and the cardiac cavities and vessels have normal appearance. The aorta arises entirely or largely from the right ventricle and the pulmonary artery arises from the left ventricle.

• Coarctation of the aorta: this is suggested by right ventricle > left ventricle; pulmonary artery much larger than aorta but a normally connected heart.

♦ See also Answer 133 in Chapter 5 (p. 350).

96 a] Ultrasound shows a $56 \times 67 \times 27$ mm predominantly hypoechoic area at the lower edge of the placenta.

b] This is probably a marginal bleed (subchorionic haematoma).

c] Future ultrasound management is to monitor the size of the haematoma, and to assess fetal well-being and growth.

♦ A decrease in the size of the haematoma is advantageous.

97 a] Ultrasound shows a single fetus. There is no obvious amniotic fluid around the fetus. There is an anterior placenta. The fetal measurements were:
BPD = 29 mm; HC = 121 mm; FL = 18 mm; AC was unobtainable. FHB was demonstrated in Fig. 6.97c.

b] The findings are consistent with anhydramnios.

♦ The lady subsequently miscarried.

98 a] Ultrasound shows a male fetus with an invisible urinary bladder. The cord insertion is lower than expected. Both kidneys were reported seen and normal, plus normal amniotic fluid.

b] Bladder extrophy is the most likely diagnosis. The differential diagnoses are omphalocele and sacrococcygeal teratoma but in both of these the urinary bladder will be seen.

c] Ultrasound would be useful to exclude hydronephrosis, secondary hydroureter and other structural abnormality, to monitor the above ultrasound findings and to assess the effect of this condition on fetal growth and well-being.

99 a] Ultrasound shows an approximately $35 \times 24 \times 40$ mm multiseptated, predominantly hypoechoic mass inferior to the left axilla on the lateral aspect of the thorax.

b] This most probably represents lymphagioma.

c] Ultrasound would be useful to exclude other structural abnormality, to monitor the above ultrasound findings and to assess the effect of this condition on fetal growth and well-being.

100 a] Fig. 6.100a and b show a $14 \times 17 \times 16$ mm irregular-in-outline hyperechoic structure outside of the heart in the right pericardium surrounded by a thin rim of fluid (pericardiac effusion). There is also an anechogenic focus.

b] Teratoma is the most likely diagnosis. Differential diagnoses are cardiac rhabdomyoma and fibroma; however, both of these are intracardiac masses.

c] Serial scans were performed to:
— monitor the ultrasound findings in Fig. 6.100a and b
— assess the effect of this condition on fetal growth and well-being
— confirm the nature of the mass
— exclude cardiac and other structural or chromosomal abnormality
— guide the necessary interventional procedure
— assess post interventional procedure effect on the mass.

d] Fig. 6.100d and e, which were obtained many weeks after the laser interventional procedure, shows that the entity is now smaller, measuring $11 \times 10 \times 18$ mm and there is now no evidence of pericardiac effusion.

101 a] The AC measurement should be repeated to reconfirm the obtained AC.

b] If the AC is still the same, the sonographer should exclude or confirm the possibility of:
— a normal small fetus (check maternal size)
— a starving fetus
— an abnormal small fetus.
The fact that the GA has been previously confirmed by LMP and ultrasound excludes the possibility of wrong date. Since no other fetal measurements were affected, the possibility of equipment fault is eliminated.

c] The AC should be interpreted together with other fetal measurements (HC: AC ratio where used) and amniotic fluid assessment. Structural abnormalities would need to be excluded whether or not the anomaly scan was done and reported previously as 'normal'.
♦ Further serial scans and Dopplers may become necessary.
♦ It has been suggested that in fetuses with an AC below the 5th centile for GA:
— 5% will be due to growth restriction, secondary to genetic disease or environmental damage
— 15% will be due to uteroplacental insufficiency or reduced placental perfusion (this group if untreated in utero are more prone to complications including perinatal death or morbidity)
— 85% would be constitutionally normally small.

A.7

Fertility

ANSWERS

1 Some of the causes of female infertility that can be evaluated by ultrasound include:
— abnormal follicles, for example polycystic ovaries (PCO) or unruptured follicle syndrome
— blocked fallopian tubes secondary to infection or endometriosis
— congenital uterine malformations, for example bicornuate uterus or hypoplastic uterus
— distortion of the endometrial cavity due to polyps or fibroids and the poor placentation that may result.

2 • Anechoic: without echo, appears as black as the fluid in the urinary bladder.
• Hyperechoic: with increased echogenicity and is white on the television monitor when compared with the myometrium and the urinary bladder.
• Isoechoic: same echogenicity as the myometrium.
• Hypoechoic: decreased echogenicity when compared with the myometrium, usually appearing darker.

3 A baseline pelvic ultrasound scan of the patient prior to fertility treatment is useful in:
— establishing the normality or otherwise of pelvic organs
— pelvic assessment which may indicate the need for further diagnostic or therapeutic procedures
— providing information which may help in deciding the appropriate treatment regimen.
— providing a base for comparison of results before, during and after treatment, for example in patients in whom a therapeutic procedure such as surgery is recommended before commencing fertility treatment
— the occasional finding of an intrauterine pregnancy with or without fetal heartbeat (FHB)
— medicolegal circumstances, although this is rarely the reason for a baseline scan.
♦ With ultrasound, the status of the pelvic anatomy could be assessed as well as the functional problems which may be of particular importance in infertility evaluation.

4 Congenital uterine malformations are rarely the primary cause of infertility but 20% of recurrent abortions are reported to be due to such development defects. Spontaneous abortion is more often associated with unicornuate, bicornuate and

septate uteri but not with arcuate or didelphic uteri. Septate uteri have the highest prevalence of habitual abortions which is thought to be due to vascular deficiencies.

- ◆ It is important to identify uterine malformations.

5 a] Criteria for monthly infertility scanning: same sonographer, same route (i.e. transvaginal or transabdominal), same ultrasound equipment (if possible), consistency in measurement and labelling of the follicles to avoid confusion.

- ◆ It may not always be possible to have the same sonographer during a treatment cycle, especially where the ultrasound facilities are not within the same fertility unit.

b] With TVS the images obtained are far superior to those from TA scan, with increased accuracy of follicular diameter measurement and visualization of the primordial follicle in much greater detail.

6 Ultrasound is useful in monitoring the number and growth of the follicles and endometrial assessment.

- ◆ In some fertility units, Doppler technique is employed to assess blood flow to the ovaries and endometrium.

7 Ultrasound is useful during fertility treatment in:

- — follicular assessment (number and size) which may indicate no response, slow response or too much response to clomifene citrate or gonadotrophins (where the ultrasound appearances and oestrogen levels are suggestive of possible ovarian hyperstimulation the patient may be coasted with ultrasound and oestrogen level monitoring prior to egg collection)
- — determining unruptured follicle syndrome
- — assessing the echopattern and thickness of the endometrium
- — assessing the blood flow to the ovaries using Doppler technique
- — egg collection using the transvaginal, transabdominal, transcervical or periurethral route
- — ultrasound-guided embryo transfer to determine proper embryo placement.
  - ◆ In some fertility units, using ultrasound is the standard procedure for all embryo transfers while in others it is reserved for difficult cases.
  - ◆ Using TVS, it has been observed that most implantation occurs with endometrial thickness of 10 mm, few occurring below 7.5 mm and none below 5 mm.

8 Ultrasound may be employed in the following prefertility treatment procedures:

- — cyst aspiration
- — uterine cavity and tubal assessment using normal saline, saline-based antibiotic preparations or other solutions of low echogenicity or echogenic contrast media-based solutions (e.g. HyCoSy).

9 Some ultrasound-identifiable conditions:

- — congenital abnormalities: bicornuate uterus, uterine didelphys, absent or rudimentary ovaries
- — pelvic masses: dermoid cyst, endometrioma, other masses, associated fluid collections

27 Secondary amenorrhoea could be the result of polycystic ovaries, weight loss, Asherman's syndrome, severe stress or psychological problems; Turner's syndrome will cause primary amenorrhoea (see also Answer 21 in Ch. A.3, p. 247).

28 OHSS is seen in association with drug therapy used for infertility treatment.

29 OHSS is divided into three grades:
   — mild OHSS whose incidence is thought to be 8–23%; presents as an elevated hormone level and enlarged ovaries on ultrasound
   — moderate OHSS whose incidence is less than 7%; presentation is as in mild OHSS but with abdominal distension, nausea, vomiting and diarrhoea
   — severe OHSS whose incidence is less than 2%; presentation is as in mild OHSS plus ascites which usually causes abdominal pain and distension. There is pleural effusion which causes shortness of breath, alteration in blood with eventual problems with clot formation and reduced blood flow to the kidneys leading to reduced urine output and renal failure if untreated.
   ◆ While OHSS can be life-threatening, 75% of women who develop OHSS are in fact pregnant.

30 The following categories of patients are more prone to OHSS:
   — women who have had a previous ultrasound history of OHSS
   — women who have polycystic ovarian syndrome
   — women who have multiple follicles
   — women with an elevated oestrogen level prior to egg collection.

31 OHSS usually presents after egg collection and embryo transfer have taken place.

32 Using ultrasound in OHSS can:
   — identify women who have polycystic ovarian syndrome
   — identify women who have multiple follicles and may be prone to developing OHSS
   — help to assess follicular measurements where the patient is being coasted prior to egg collection
   — help to assess ovarian size and the presence of ascites in patients who have developed OHSS following egg collection and embryo transfer.

33 From the exact time of ovulation, the times when embyronic structures (e.g. gestational sac, yolk sac, fetal pole, FHB) will be visible on ultrasound can then be calculated.

34 It has been suggested that transmigration of the ovum is an important factor in ectopic pregnancies with a corpus luteal cyst noted on the opposite side of the ectopic pregnancy in 13–23% of cases. The presence of a corpus luteal cyst does not help in terms of localizing an ectopic pregnancy.

35 An abnormal bleeding or implantational bleeding at the expected time of a period can be mistaken for a normal period. Although pelvic pain and tenderness are non-specific signs of gynaecological problems, a pelvic ultrasound might be beneficial in such cases.

36 Sliding organ sign is the ability of the uterus or ovary to slide away from the adjacent pelvic structure when the transvaginal probe is gently used to push it away and the space created could be imaged under real-time ultrasound. Failure

of the ovary or the uterus to slide past each other when pressure is applied may be suggestive of adhesions which can be a cause of infertility.

37 • Male factors in infertility:
   — congenital abnormalities such as cryptorchidism (undescended testes), Klinefelter's syndrome (XXY), Kallmann's syndrome and Kartagener's (immotile cilia) syndrome
   — previous scrotal or testicular injury, including vasectomy, causing significant antisperm antibodies
   — no sperm
   — absent or blocked sperm duct
   — poor quality or quantity of sperm
   — erectile impotence
   — male genital tract infection
   — drugs, especially anabolic steroids
   — idiopathic
   — testicular failure following chemotherapy
   — retrograde ejaculation following prostatic surgery, urinary bladder neck surgery or problems with the nerve supply to the urinary bladder neck.

• Female factors in infertility:
   — congenital abnormalities which may affect the uterus and/or ovary
   — a woman who has never menstruated in her life due to a genetic defect (e.g. Turner's syndrome)
   — early cessation of menstruation (early menopause)
   — cervical factor in which the cervical environment in the woman is very hostile to her husband's sperm and so kills them off
   — ovarian disorders such as polycystic or multicystic ovaries, polycystic ovarian disease
   — ovarian cysts of all types such as endometrioma, dermoid (cystic teratoma)
   — ovulation defects (e.g. hyperprolactinaemia)
   — tubal problems such as blocked tubes, or fluid- or pus-filled tubes (hydrosalpinx, pyosalpinx)
   — pelvic inflammatory disease (PID)
   — space-occupying lesions in the endometrial cavity such as fibroids or polyps.
   ◆ Tubal blockage may be secondary to ascending infection (e.g. secondary to sexually transmitted disease), descending infection from other sites in the peritoneal cavity (e.g. from the appendix), following a sterilization procedure or other previous abdominal surgery.

• Combined factors: subfertility may be due to some factors in the man *and* the woman (e.g. low sperm count and polycystic ovary).

• Unexplained factors: when after the battery of tests no medical cause can be found in the couple for subfertility yet the woman is unable to conceive.

• Incompatibility factors: very rarely a situation in which there is incompatibility between the sperm and the egg.

- ◆ Ovum donation is useful in patients who:
  - — are carriers of an inheritable disorder or genetic disease (e.g. cystic fibrosis, thalassaemia, haemophilia, sickle cell disease, Duchenne muscular dystrophy or Tay–Sachs disease) who wish to avoid the same in their offspring
  - — suffer from premature ovarian failure
  - — do not have ovaries but have a uterus
  - — have suffered ovarian damage following radiotherapy or chemotherapy treatments or surgery
  - — unfortunately habitually miscarry
  - — have many failed IVF treatments, either due to poor ovarian response or with apparently normal eggs which fail to fertilize (number will depend on unit protocol).
- *Assisted hatching*: as in IVF except that in order to enhance the chances of implantation, a small hole is made in the shell of the embryo by a localized exposure of the embryo shell to an acidified solution to remove the zona pellucida of the embryo.
- *Subzonal insemination (SUZI)*: sperm is aspirated by fine needle and deposited into the perivitelline space of the oocyte.
  - ◆ There are no data to suggest that children born from ICSI or SUZI have a higher abnormality rate than those conceived naturally.
  - ◆ Other forms of fertility treatment include *surrogacy* and *egg sharing in a fertility centre*.
39 Factors influencing choice of fertility treatment:
  - Sperm – availability, quality, quantity and motility
  - Uterus – presence or absence
  - Eggs – availability, quality and quantity
  - Female age
  - Ovary – presence or absence and if functional
  - Fallopian tubes – absence, presence, patency and state (e.g. hydro- or pyosalpinx)
  - Inherited or genetically transferable disease which the couple want to avoid
  - Available fertility treatment options in the fertility centre
  - Costs – where the patient has to pay for some or all of the following: drugs, medical fees, accommodation, transportation, i.e. affordability to the couple.
  - ◆ Often the available fertility treatment options in any set-up are primarily influenced by laboratory facilities, staff expertise and the HFEA licence given.
40 Medical terminology relating to aspects of fertility:
  - Azoospermia – no spermatozoa in the ejaculate
  - Aspermia – no ejaculate
  - Asthenozoospermia – fewer than 50% spermatozoa with forward progression
  - Teratospermia – fewer than 50% spermatozoa with normal morphology
  - Normozoospermia – normal ejaculate as defined by the World Health Organization (WHO)

- Oligospermia – sperm concentration fewer than 20 million per ml
- Infertility – the absolute absence of the ability to conceive
- Subfertility – the failure to conceive after 1 year of normal coitus or reduced likelihood of conception or sterility when investigations show that the couple has a low chance of conceiving
- Primary infertility – no previous pregnancy in history
- Secondary infertility – previous pregnancy did occur.
- ◆ The terms infertility and subfertility are sometime used interchangeably.

41 Infertility investigations:
- Ultrasound scan – see Answers 1 and 3 on page 390.
- Laboratory tests to assess:
  — follicle stimulating hormone (FSH) is observed to be high in patients with primary or secondary ovarian failure
  — luteinizing hormone (LH) is observed to be high in patients with PCO who are also at risk of miscarriage
  — prolactin level, as high prolactin can suppress ovulation thus causing infertility
  — Day 21 progesterone may be monitored over three or four cycles to confirm or exclude an irregular ovulatory cycle
  — chlamydia (sexually transmitted disease) screening test for tubal problems (it is suggested that many pelvic infections are due to chlamydia infection)
  — rubella immunity as pregnancy should be avoided for 3 months following immunization.
- Hysterosalpingography or transvaginal sonosalpingography – to assess the uterine cavity and exclude any tubal pathology (see also Answer 53, p. 403).
- Postcoital test – a sample of the secretions from the posterior fornix is taken following sexual intercourse to assess the availability of living sperm and its quantity. *This test may no longer be necessary as the nature of secretions from the cervix will not be of importance for couples who choose to have fertility treatment such as artificial insemination, IVF or ICSI. (In some units this is combined with ultrasound scan to confirm that ovulation has taken place.)
- Laparoscopy – to assess tubal patency (laparoscopy and dye test) and any underlying pelvic pathology, including uterine adhesions and fibroids, and could be applied therapeutically, using laser or diathermy, in treating adhesions, endometriosis or polycystic ovaries.
- Hysteroscopy – for excluding intrauterine pathology such as polyps and for assessing the shape of the cavity.
- ◆ Which of the above tests is done and when will depend on many factors as well as the departmental protocol.

42 a] Hyperprolactinaemia is a condition whereby there is excessive prolactin that sometimes causes the non-lactating breast to secrete milk. A high prolactin level can suppress ovulation and cause infertility. It is estimated that about 5% of cases will present with visual field defect in cases of microscopic prolactinoma.

- ◆ Prolactinoma. A mildly increased prolactin level may be due to recent general physical examination, specific breast examination or stress.
- ◆ Hyperprolactinaemia causes secondary amenorrhoea.
- ◆ Hyperprolactinaemia may be due to pituitary adenoma, non-functioning 'disconnection' tumour in the region of the hypothalamus or pituitary which disrupts the inhibitory influence of dopamine on prolactin secretion, hypothyroidism, some drugs and PCO syndrome.

b] Diagnostic tests for hyperprolactinaemia include:
- — laboratory test to assess the level of serum prolactin
- — thyroid function test (hypothyroidism is associated with hyperprolactinaemia)
- — CT or MRI scan of the pituitary fossa to rule out a prolactinoma (pituitary tumour).

43 a] ◆ *Short protocol*: the downregulation is not complete before the gonadotrophin injection starts. There is therefore a large boost of FSH from the extra FSH available due to the nasal spray displacing the stored FSH from the pituitary gland. In the short protocol, the patient starts using the nasal spray on Day 1 of her cycle. She adds fertility injections on Days 3–4, provided the scan findings are satisfactory, and continues both medications daily. Her response to medication is monitored with ultrasound, with or without laboratory tests, until she is deemed ready for egg collection, at which time an ovulatory dose of hCG is administered in the night and egg collection scheduled for 36 hours later.

- ◆ *Long protocol*: downregulation is started on Day 21 of the previous cycle prior to starting IVF or ICSI (i.e. luteal phase in a Day 21 protocol) and continued into the treatment cycle. When an adequate pituitary response has been achieved, daily gonadotrophin injections are added to the regimen, provided the scan findings are satisfactory, and continues both medications daily. Her response to the medication is monitored with ultrasound, with or without laboratory tests, until she is deemed ready for egg collection, at which time an ovulatory dose of hCG is administered in the night and egg collection scheduled for 36 hours later. *Alternatively*:

  Downregulation is started on Day 1 of the treatment cycle (i.e. early follicular phase in a Day 1 protocol) and continued until an adequate pituitary response has been achieved, when daily gonadotrophin injections are added to the regimen, provided the scan findings are satisfactory, and continues both medications daily. Her response to the medication is monitored with ultrasound, with or without laboratory tests, until she is deemed ready for egg collection, at which time an ovulatory dose of hCG is administered in the night and egg collection scheduled for 36 hours later.

- ◆ Pituitary suppression could be assessed by measuring the serum LH or the serum oestradiol or by measuring the thickness of the endometrium on ultrasound.

b] The short protocol is useful in women with a previous poor response to fertility treatment, and in older women because their ovarian reserve is generally reduced and they require less suppression. The long protocol, therefore, may oversuppress them.

c] Advantages and disadvantages of the short and long protocols

Protocol	Advantages	Disadvantages
Short protocol	Ability to confine fertility treatment to same menstrual cycle Fewer gonadotrophin injections needed therefore less patient drug cost	Not very flexible May not be as successful as the long protocol
Long protocol	Greater number of eggs and embryos Maximum degree of flexibility with the cycle Better success rate than in short protocol	Increased patient drug cost as the medication duration is longer

d] Likely times for performing the ultrasound scans:
  — short protocol: Days 3–4 and 7–8 days later**
  — ultrashort protocol: Days 3–4 and 11–12 and**
  — long Day 1 protocol: Days 3, 10, 17–18 and**
  — long Day 21 protocol: Days 3–4, 10–12 and**.
  ** Subsequent scans are individually decided by the clinician. These are mostly dependent on the ovarian response.

e] Days 2–3 in a short protocol, Days 3–4 in a long Day 21 or long Day 1 protocol, and Day 10 in a long Day 1 protocol are the best times to assess the endometrial thickness and check that the ovaries are in their resting state (quiescent), indicating a good response to the luteinizing hormone-releasing hormone (LH-RH) analogue before commencing the gonadotrophin injections.

Seven days after commencing the gonadotrophin injections in all the protocols is the best time to assess ovarian response to the fertility drugs. Ovarian response may also influence endometrial thickness.

♦ Subsequent scans are used to assess follicular development and endometrial thickness so that egg collection can be best timed.
♦ LH-RH is usually discontinued prior to the late night hCG injection.
♦ Should the patient shows ultrasound signs of a possible OHSS then she may be coasted.
♦ Day 1 is taken to be the first full day of menstrual bleed in the cycle.
♦ It is not uncommon for a few ladies to develop ovarian cysts while on the LH-RH analogue before starting the fertility injections.
♦ See also Answer 7 on page 391.

44 Profasi is an injection which is given 2–3 days following egg collection while Cyclogest is a suppository given to prepare the uterus for a potential pregnancy. Either is prescribed by the clinician for the patient.

♦ hCG or progesterone are given after embryo transfer as luteal support. After downregulation, the central system does not produce luteinizing hormone to stimulate the follicle to produce progesterone which is vital for the endometrium to thicken and facilitate implantation. Therefore hCG, which is similar to LH, is given to stimulate the follicle to produce progesterone.
♦ In patients with OHSS or PCO, an elevated hCG level will have side effects, thus the correct dose of progesterone will have to be given instead.

45 The LH-RH analogue is meant to suppress the hormones from the pituitary gland of the brain which would normally stimulate the ovary in approximately 10–14 days after starting the injection. The normal functions of the ovaries would then be 'switched off', thus permitting better control over the recruitment of the follicles in response to the administered fertility injections as well as preventing a preovulatory surge which in turn will prevent spontaneous ovulation.

  ◆ The currently available LH-RH analogues include buserelin, nafarelin, goserelin and leuprorelin acetate. These could be administered as a daily subcutaneous injection, nasal spray or as a depot (long-acting) injection.
  ◆ The currently available gonadotrophin injections include follitropin alfa (Gonal-F) and urofollitropin (Metrodin High Purity).

46 a] Ultrasound shows a 51.4×55.9 mm predominantly cystic area with areas of low level echoes within it.

  b] Left endometrioma is the most likely diagnosis.

  c] Endometriosis is thought to be present in 5–20% of women of reproductive age and a cause of infertility in 5–15% of all cases of infertility and in 30% of cases in which no other significant abnormality is found.

  d] Differential diagnosis is haemorrhagic corpus luteal cyst. With a corpus luteal cyst, progressive changes of the internal echo pattern will be observed due to fibrinolysis of the blood over a period of time. Such cysts usually disappear with menstruation and do not cause infertility. Scanning the woman in another phase of her menstrual cycle will confirm this.

  ◆ Ovarian endometrioma may be cystic, polycystic, mixed or solid in appearance. Physical symptoms include dysmenorrhoea which often starts some years after pain-free menstruation, infertility, dyspareunia and chronic pelvic pain.

47 a] There are two types of unicornuate uterus: with a rudimentary horn and without a rudimentary horn.

  b] It is important to know whether or not there is a rudimentary horn, if this horn is functional and lined by endometrium, whether or not the horn has a cavity and if there is any communication with the developed unicornuate horn. It has been suggested that there is an increased risk of endometriosis and pelvic adhesions when there is no communication between a rudimentary horn that has an endometrial cavity and a unicornuate uterus. This is said to be due to outflow tract obstruction.

48 Severe vaginitis, pelvic inflammatory disease (PID), painful adnexal masses such as giant posterior fibroid, ectopic pregnancy and vaginismus may make transvaginal ultrasound painful.

49 Protective covers for the transvaginal probe:

  • The glove: thicker than condoms and it has been suggested that the tearing of holes occurs less frequently than with condoms. For some individuals, it could be more time consuming and difficult to use because of its five fingers.
  • The non-spermicidal condom: easier to use but more prone to tearing of holes.
  • The specialized probe cover: there are specially designed probe covers that can be used but it has been implied that there is no added advantage to using them over the glove and the condom and there is an additional cost implication.

- Whichever protective cover is used, it should be checked before use for a leak.
- It is good practice to check with the patient before commencing TVS for her sensitivity to latex and to have available a non-latex alternative.
- Sonographers should be aware of their own sensitivity to latex, the symptoms of latex sensitivity and what to do if such should occur.
- It is estimated that latex allergies are rare, affecting an estimated 1–3% of the population.
- Decontamination of the probe between patients and sterilization at set times in line with the manufacturer's instructions are advisable.

50 a] Ultrasound shows an anteverted uterus with a thickened endometrium measuring 11 mm.
   b] Uterine blood vessels constitute the hypoechoic structure.
   - Uterine blood vessels are easiest to visualize 1–2 weeks after the onset of the last menstrual period (LMP) and are most difficult to image before or during the menstrual period. This is thought to be due to the vasodilating action of oestrogen on the uterus in the mid-cycle, resulting in an increase in the blood supply, and a vasoconstricting hormonal influence during the late luteal phase of the menstrual cycle.

51 a] Ultrasound shows a transverse scan of the uterus with two endometriums, each 14 mm thick, suggesting a bicornuate uterus. Some fluid is demonstrated in the POD.
   - A bicornuate uterus is thought to be due to the incomplete fusion of the caudal portion of the müllerian ducts.
   b] Though not a cause for infertility, patients with bicornuate uterus are said to have a higher rate of spontaneous abortions, preterm labour and malpresentation.
   c] Ultrasound-guided artificial insemination or embryo transfer will be beneficial where it is not a common practice.

52 a] Ultrasound shows a 12 mm echogenic mass within the endometrium. This possibly represents a polyp.
   - The differential diagnosis is an intracavity myoma which is likely to be seen with posterior shadows.
   b] Polyps have been associated with infertility. They are believed to affect implantation of the conceptus in the same way that an intrauterine contraceptive device (IUCD) affects implantation. They also account for 6.8% of menometrorrhagia in women of reproductive age. They are best seen during the late proliferative phase but can be seen in the periovulatory and secretory phases.
   c] By instilling some fluid (e.g. normal saline) into the cavity under ultrasound control will help in assessing this structure.
   d] A polyp is a pedunculated tumour of the mucous membrane.
   - The pathology report confirmed that it was a polyp.

53 The advantages of assessing the uterine cavity and tubes with ultrasound and instillation of fluid instead of using the conventional HSG include:
   — it does not use ionizing radiation and is potentially safer
   — it can be done early in the menstrual cycle without risk to any ensuing pregnancy

— generally there is no need for analgesia
— imaging and evaluating the ovaries, the uterine wall, cervix and adnexal structures can be done at the same time
— it is potentially more convenient and less expensive
— idiosyncrasy to the contrast agent cannot be expected
— the investigation could be performed on an ambulatory basis as a screening procedure
— it may be used to assess tubal status after microsurgery for reanastomosis and it is clearly indicated in patients with a history of reactions to iodinated contrast medium.

♦ The patient may experience some mild transient discomfort and many patients claim that this discomfort is less than what they experience with the conventional HSG.

♦ It has been suggested that transvaginal sonosalpingography does not provide an accurate assessment of intrauterine and tubal anatomy. The technique is dependent on the experience of the sonographer in evaluating the images which are quite different from the classical findings, especially in the assessment of both tubal structures.

♦ In one particular department, a woman is prepared for HSG as follows: she is to phone to let the department know when her menstrual period comes on. HSG is not done on days 1–10 to avoid extravasation of the contrast medium. No sex is allowed in the HSG cycle until after the examination and the patient is required to sign a form confirming this before the examination.

54 Some of the reported fluid materials used in ultrasound-guided uterine and tubal assessment include sterile isotonic saline, sterile water, physiologic saline solution which contains crystalline penicillin and hydrocortisone, and contrast medium SHU 454 (Echovist; Schering, Berlin, Germany).

♦ Choice of fluid used varies from one department to another.

♦ Use of SHU 454 is contraindicated in patients who have galactosaemia because of the saccharide galactose content of the echo contrast medium. However, it is suggested that the sticky nature of the echo contrast medium is able to outline submucous fibroids well enough to assess the contours of the fibroids within the uterine cavity.

55 a] Ultrasound shows a retroverted uterus with a posterior fibroid (leiomyoma) measuring 30×34 mm which is anteriorly displacing the cavity.

b] It is thought that interference with reproductive capability is most likely a function of the size and location of the leiomyoma. They can impair the patency of the reproductive tract by occluding the cervical canal or the intramural portion of the fallopian tubes. They can distort the isthmic or ampullary portion of the oviduct and interfere with the relationship of this structure to the ovary, causing changes in oocyte transport. The enlarged and distorted uterus may result in poor transport of the sperm.

♦ The ultrasound appearance of a fibroid may also show randomly distributed calcifications or calcifications at the periphery outlining it. Although not thought to be a common cause of infertility, fibroids are said to be seen in 40% of women over 35 years old. It has also been noted that fibroids are more common in dark skinned women.

56 Ultrasound could be used to assess accurately the specific size and location of leiomyomas and to monitor the growth of small leiomyomas.

57 A submucous fibroid may cause 1st or 2nd trimester abortion, premature labour and abnormal fetal presentation. It may distort uterine cavity contour, thus impacting greatly on reproductive outcome. It may hinder endometrial nutrition which may result in poor placentation and intrauterine growth retardation.

58 a] Ultrasound shows a predominantly hyperechoic area within the endometrium, possibly a polyp.
   b] The aim of the saline introduction was to assess the cavity and determine the exact location of the mass in relation to the cavity and the likely nature of the mass.
   c] Ultrasound shows some fluid outlining the same mass but with posterior acoustic shadowing. This is probably a submucous fibroid.
   • The mass is a fibroid within the endometrium, which was confirmed at surgery.

59 Ultrasound is rarely used following failed fertility treatment except in instances where the patient has symptoms of OHSS which is being monitored.

60 Ultrasound following a successful treatment cycle:
   • 2 weeks after embryo transfer a pregnancy test is done. If the pregnancy test result is positive a scan will be done 2 weeks later to:
     — confirm intrauterine pregnancy or otherwise
     — confirm the number of gestational sac(s)
     — if seen, confirm FHB
     — assess the ovaries, any cysts within, any associated pelvic fluid and any other previously noted mass(es).
   • 2 weeks after the first scan, another ultrasound scan is done to:
     — check that the pregnancy(ies) is ongoing by checking FHB
     — check the number of fetus(es) with FHB
     — check that gestational age is equal to dates
     — assess the ovaries, any cysts within, any associated pelvic fluid and any other previously noted mass(es).
   ♦ In cases of OHSS with pregnancy, ultrasound may be used to assess the OHSS.
   ♦ This is a protocol in use in one particular fertility unit; it may differ in other units.

61 a] Ultrasound shows at least nine follicles in the right ovary and four follicles in the left ovary, many of which are greater than 10 mm and a 7.7 mm endometrium.
   b] This is referred to as a flare-up reaction to the use of the analogue.

62 a] Ultrasound shows a longitudinal section of the liver and right kidney. Abundant ascites is present outlining some bowel loops.
   b] Enlarged ovaries with multiple cysts and ascites may also be found in this pelvis.
   c] This is severe ovarian hyperstimulation syndrome (OHSS).

63 a] Ultrasound shows an ovary with at least four hypoechoic areas, possibly follicles, as well as another $\geq 20 \times 30$ mm low level echo area within which is a hyperechoic area measuring $\geq 10 \times 20$ mm.

b] Ultrasound appearance is suggestive of a dermoid cyst. This was confirmed at surgery.

- ◆ Dermoids have many sonographic patterns depending on the components of the cyst. Dermoids tend to occur in young women.

c] It is thought that interference with reproductive capability is most likely if the dermoid is large and is compressing the ovary, thus affecting ovulation from that side. Where the fallopian tube gets stuck to a dermoid it could become stretched as the dermoid gets larger. It could leak without symptoms and cause peritonitis and adhesions. Adhesions are known to be one of the causes of infertility.

- ◆ It has been suggested that a dermoid cyst be removed before embarking on fertility treatment so as to enhance ovarian response.

64 a] Ultrasound shows a 105×77 mm hypoechoic irregular tubular structure.

b] In view of the fact that the structure is hypoechoic with no low echoes demonstrated within it, this is likely to be a right hydrosalpinx (confirmed at surgery performed pretreatment).

c] It is believed that fluid may leak from the hydrosalpinx into the uterine cavity physically flushing out the embryos from the uterus, and thus preventing implantation, or that the hydrosalpinx fluid may have toxic effects on the embryos.

d] The available options for treating hydrosalpinx are:

- — ignoring it and proceeding with treatment
- — salpingectomy before commencing treatment
- — draining the hydrosalpinx during egg collection
- — laparoscopic tubal clipping of the right tube.
- ◆ Hydrosalpinx is prone to reaccumulating fluid during ovarian stimulation. If the chosen treatment option is to drain it, this is preferably done during egg collection with antibiotic cover.

65 a] Ultrasound shows a spiral, 120 mm tubular structure with low level echoes within it. The features are suggestive of a right pyosalpinx.

b] Ultrasound shows a 27×45 mm low level echo area on the right. The right ovary was not seen separate from this structure. This probably represents a right endometrioma.

- ◆ See also Answer 46 on page 402.

66 a] Ultrasound shows many peripheral tiny cysts in the ovary with a 'string-of-pearls' appearance and hyperechoic central stroma.

b] Polycystic ovary is the most likely diagnosis.

c] Women with polycystic ovaries tend to have irregular menstrual periods or no periods at all; they may be anovulatory; pregnancy is more difficult to achieve, probably due to irregular ovulation, and they may have poor quality oocytes. Those with high circulating levels of luteinizing hormone are prone to miscarriage.

d] There may be hyperstimulation, or the follicles may take a longer time to mature or not grow to the expected size.

67 a] Ultrasound shows a possible gestational ring outside the uterus

     b] Ectopic pregnancy is the most likely diagnosis (confirmed at surgery).

68 a] Ectopic pregnancy is more prevalent in women:
  - with a history of previous ectopic pregnancy (it is estimated that the recurrence of ectopic is 10% of all ectopic pregnancies)
  - with tubal problems, congenital tubal anomalies or previous tubal surgery (e.g. tubal sterilization, peritubal adhesions from surgery or infection)
  - with a history of PID
  - with endometriosis
  - who conceive while wearing an IUCD
  - who conceive while taking the progesterone-only pill
  - who are in assisted conception programmes.
  - ◆ Bleeding occurs in about 50–75% of cases of ectopic pregnancy. Incidence is about 0.5–1% of all pregnancies but it is responsible for 10% of all maternal deaths. Overall, 97.5% of ectopic pregnancies occur in the fallopian tubes, 0.7% in the ovaries and 1.8% elsewhere in the abdominal cavity.

     b] A heterotopic pregnancy is one in which an intrauterine pregnancy coexists with an ectopic pregnancy.

     c] Incidence of heterotopic pregnancy is 1 in 4000 to 1 in 30 000.
  - ◆ Patients undergoing an IVF programme are said to be at a higher risk of heterotopic pregnancy with an incidence as high as 1 in 100. This is thought to be due to the presence of underlying pelvic disease such as blocked tubes. Careful examination of the adnexa should therefore be performed to rule out this possibility in patients receiving ovulatory drugs.

     d] Ectopic pregnancy can present with pelvic pain, pelvic tenderness, abnormal vaginal bleeding, missed or late period and adnexal mass, plus cardiovascular symptoms of instability such as dizziness, fainting, shortness of breath, anaemia and/or hypotension.

- ◆ A history of normal pregnancy or intrauterine pregnancy does not rule out an ectopic pregnancy. An abnormal bleeding or implantational bleeding at the expected time of a period may be mistaken for a normal menstrual period.

69 a] Ultrasound shows an intrauterine gestational sac with a fetal pole measuring 12 mm and a yolk sac.

     b] The image on the left of Fig. 7.69b is a B-mode (brightness mode) image display, while the image on the right is an M-mode (movement mode) image display.

     c] The ultrasound finding is of an intrauterine pregnancy with FHB and a crown–rump length (CRL) of 12 mm.

     d] The ultrasound findings do not correlate to the LMP. Going by the known LMP the fetus should be 19 weeks gestational age (GA), but was found to be 7 weeks and 4 days using the departmental chart. This gestational age discrepancy was no surprise in view of patient's known irregular menstrual cycle.

- ◆ Since an ongoing pregnancy is always an unexpected finding in a couple seeking fertility treatment at the initial consultation, the departmental protocol will influence communicating the scan findings to the couple.
- ◆ See Answer 3 on page 390.

70 Thickening of the endometrium cannot be used to diagnose pregnancy because the same appearance can be:
— seen in a late phase of the menstrual cycle
— seen in a very early intrauterine pregnancy, i.e. before the gestational sac can be resolved
— seen as a decidual reaction in association with ectopic pregnancy
— confused with retained products of conception within the uterine cavity.

71 a] Ultrasound shows an anteverted uterus with an endometrium which is 12 mm thick. The right ovary appears normal. There was a circular hypoechoic area measuring 27×27 mm in the left ovary with no echoes seen within it. This is probably a cyst.
b] The cyst in the left ovary was most likely to have caused the lack of her period.
c] The cyst is possibly producing oestrogen which is causing the endometrial thickening and inhibiting the onset of menstruation in this patient.

72 A Day 3 scan is requested:
— to check whether or not the endometrial lining has been completely shed in the menstruation before commencing fertility drugs
— to confirm or otherwise that the ovaries are quiet (resting)
— to assess other pelvic structures.
◆ The fact that a patient has bled for 3 days does not rule out a thickened endometrium or the presence of an ovarian cyst.

73 Ultrasound is used in the postcoital test to:
— assess the growth of the dominant follicle
— determine whether ovulation has occurred
— check the presence of mucus in the cervical canal.

74 a] Ultrasound shows two gestational sacs. Sac 1 is normal in size and has a fetal pole of 13 mm. Sac 2 is smaller than expected and has a yolk sac and a fetal pole of approximately 4 mm.
b] Sac 1 is ongoing but the ultrasound appearances of sac 2 are suggestive of a missed abortion.

75 a] Ultrasound shows two gestational sacs in the uterus (dichorionic diamniotic sacs). The posterior sac has a yolk sac and a fetal pole. There is a 13×15 mm posterior fibroid.
b] There are various maternal and fetal risks associated with multiple pregnancy. Although multiple pregnancy is estimated at 1 in 75 deliveries in hospitals, they account for 10% of perinatal deaths, with the perinatal mortality rate for twins being quoted as 10 times higher than that for singletons. Twin pregnancies also suffer from a higher rate of late abortion and late neonatal and infant death.
◆ The use of assisted reproduction techniques increases the risk of multiple pregnancy to 10% with clomiphene citrate and up to 40% with gonadotrophin usage. The twinning rate with IVF is dependent on the number of embryos replaced within the uterus.
◆ Up to three embryos are allowed for transfer by the HFEA guidelines in the UK at present. The number of embryos allowed for transfer may be different in other countries.

- The role of ultrasound in monitoring multiple pregnancies includes diagnosis, determination of chorionicity, monitoring of fetal growth, detection of discordant growth and detecting fetal abnormalities.

76 Ultrasound shows three intrauterine gestational sacs.

- Until the fetal heartbeats are seen the number of fetuses with FHB cannot be confirmed, therefore implying rescanning the patient in another 2 weeks or according to departmental protocol. The number of gestational sacs does not necessarily correlate with the number of fetuses.

77 a] Ultrasound shows an intrauterine gestational sac. To the left of the sac is an echopoor area.

   b] The echopoor area may be an implantational bleed.

   c] The echopoor area could be reassessed by rescanning the patient at a later date (e.g. 2 weeks later).

   - The pregnancy went well with no significant problems.

78 Luteal phase defect is asynchrony in the development of the endometrium that can lead to inadequate endometrial preparation at the time of implantation. It is reported in 1–3% of infertile couples, usually with recurrent pregnancy loss.

79 An immature endometrium can prevent implantation or be inadequate in maintaining an early gestation.

80 a] In Fig. 7.80a there are many peripheral tiny follicles of less than 10 mm with a string-of-pearls appearance and hyperechoic central stroma. In Fig. 7.80b there are again many tiny follicles of less than 10 mm but these are scattered throughout the ovary, appearing like a honeycomb.

   b] Fig. 7.80a demonstrates a polycystic ovary; Fig. 7.80b demonstrates a multicystic ovary which is thought to be a variant of polycystic ovary. This ultrasound appearance may be common in young women who, in the course of dieting or losing a lot of weight, experience amenorrhoea.

81 a] • *Polycystic ovary* describes the ultrasound appearance of the ovary. Such ovaries are seen with at least 10 peripheral immature follicles less than 10 mm. The ovary may or may not be enlarged. 20–25% of women are thought to have polycystic ovaries without having any symptoms.

   - *Polycystic ovarian disease* describes the ultrasound appearance of the ovary plus endocrinological findings. The ovary is usually enlarged $> 8 \text{ cm}^3$ in two-thirds of cases with multiple immature follicles of less than 10 mm, it may be isoechoic or hypoechoic, there is anovulation and the endometrium appears atypical or resting follicular. Clinically there may be obesity, hirsutism, amenorrhoea or menometrorrhagia, infertility and oligomenorrhoea. There is an elevation in serum LH, increased LH:FSH ratio of 3 or greater, and/or elevated serum testosterone and/or androstenedione.

   - Endometrial cancer, although rare, is possible in patients with PCOD. This is thought to be due to the thickened endometrium in women who have few or absent periods. The endometrium should be carefully assessed on ultrasound for thickening or irregularity.

   - A normal-sized ovary does not exclude PCOD.

    d] Future ultrasound management includes tapping the pleural effusion and ascites under ultrasound control and later confirming the location of the gestational sac, how many, and confirming FHB as well as follow-up assessment of these ultrasound findings.

♦ See also Answers 29–31 on page 394.

REFERENCE

Dodson M G 1995 Transvaginal ultrasound, 2nd edn. Churchill Livingstone, New York

Winston R, Salter-Murison B (eds) 1991 Infertility. Update Postgraduate Centre series. Reed Healthcare Communications, Sutton, Surrey

SECTION 3

SECTION CONTENTS

Chart 2 Growth chart (not drawn to scale)

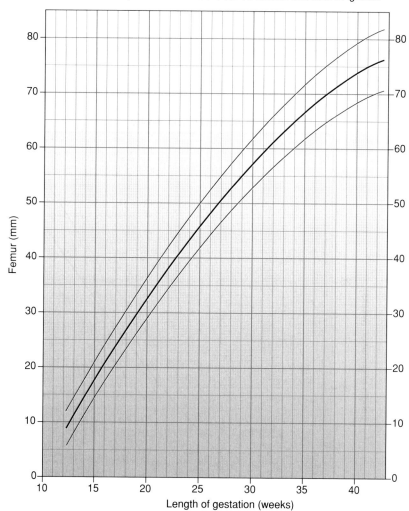

Growth chart—5th, 50th and 95th centiles. To assess fetal size for growth

Chart 3 Biparietal diameter (Question 6.48a)

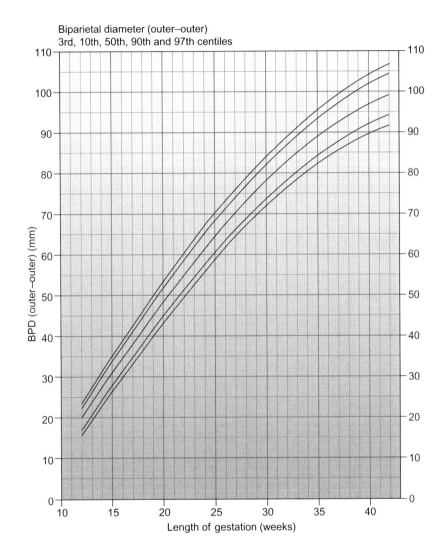

Biparietal diameter (outer–outer)
3rd, 10th, 50th, 90th and 97th centiles

BPD (outer–outer) (mm)

Length of gestation (weeks)

Chart 6 Femur length (Question 6.48a)

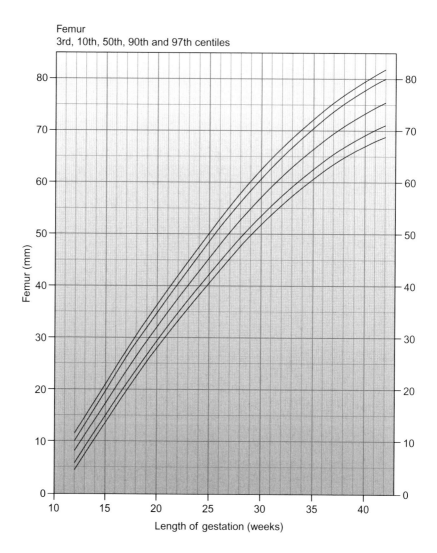

Femur
3rd, 10th, 50th, 90th and 97th centiles

Chart 7 Femur length – dating chart (Question 6.75a)

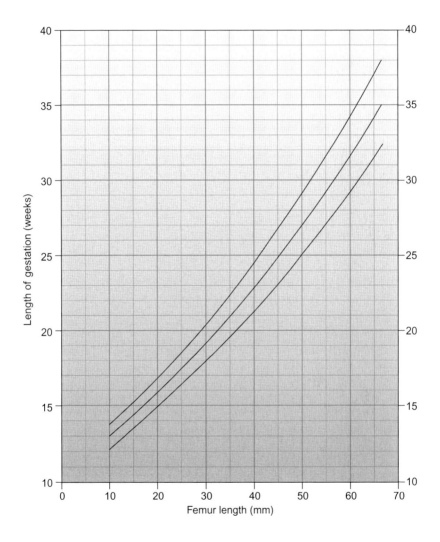

Chart 8 Transverse cerebellar diameter – dating chart (Question 6.75a)

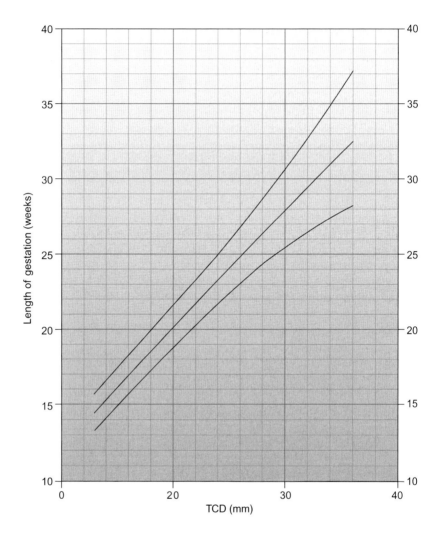

Chart 9 Head circumference – dating chart (Question 6.75a)

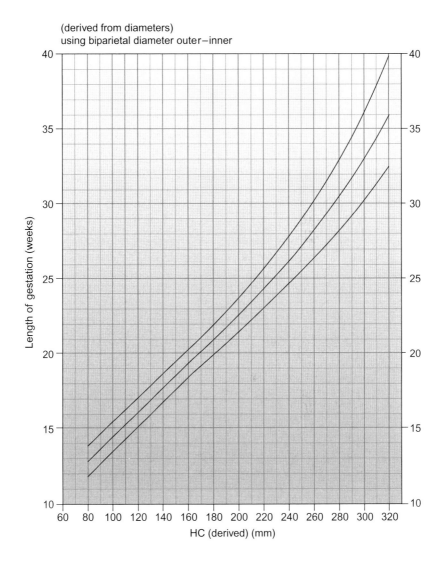

(derived from diameters)
using biparietal diameter outer–inner

Chart 10 Biparietal diameter – dating chart (Question 6.75a)

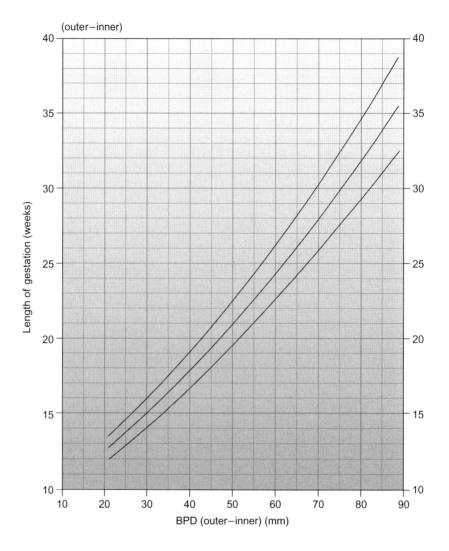

Chart 11 Head circumference (Question 6.76a)

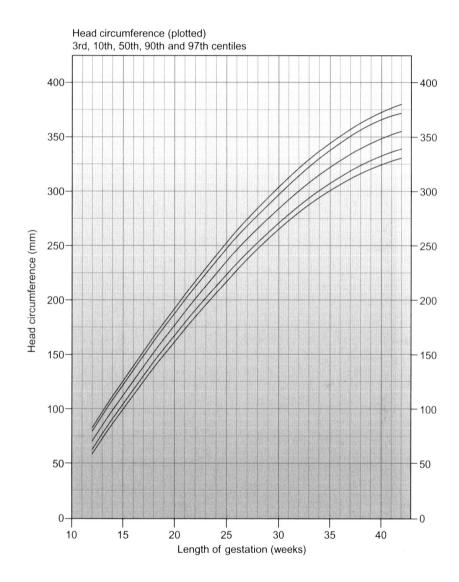

Head circumference (plotted)
3rd, 10th, 50th, 90th and 97th centiles

Chart 20 Biparietal diameter – dating chart (Answer 6.75a)

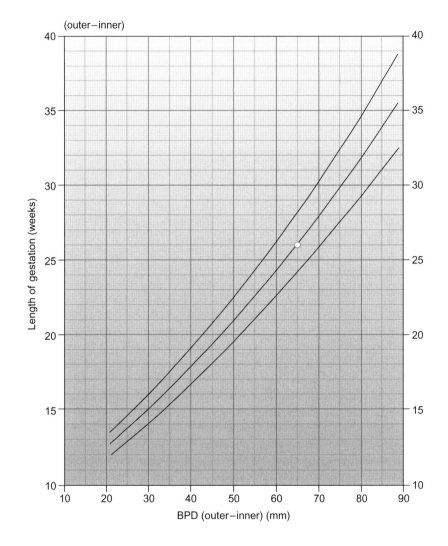

Chart 21 Head circumference (Answer 6.76a)

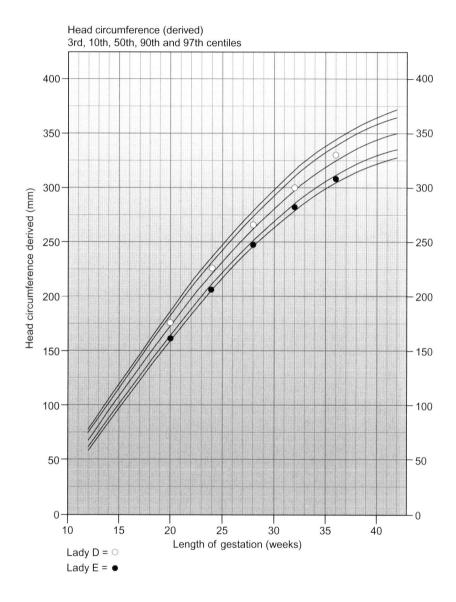

Head circumference (derived)
3rd, 10th, 50th, 90th and 97th centiles

Lady D = ○
Lady E = ●

about such treatments, and provide detailed advice and information to the public. The Publications section offers links to patient guides, code of practice and information leaflets.

The Miscarriage Association
c/o Clayton Hospital
Northgate
Wakefield
West Yorkshire WF1 3JS
Tel (helpline): 01924 200799; admin: 01924 200795
Scottish helpline: 0131 334 8883 (answerphone with names of local contacts)
http://www.miscarriageassociation.org.uk

The Miscarriage Association publishes leaflets, fact sheets and audiotapes and also has on-line information about miscarriage, ectopic pregnancy and molar pregnancy, including what is currently known about possible causes and the different treatments available. They can provide information on the hospital provision of specialist services relating to pregnancy loss and maintain a directory of other organizations which may also be of help.

Royal College of Midwives
15 Mansfield Street
London W1G 9NH
Tel: 020 7312 3538
http://www.rcm.org.uk/

The Royal College of Midwives (RCM) is the only trade union and professional organization run by midwives for midwives. It is the voice of midwifery, providing excellence in professional leadership, education, influence and representation for and on behalf of midwives. The RCM produces information and advice on a wide range of midwifery issues.

Royal College of Obstetricians and Gynaecologists
27 Sussex Place
Regents Park
London NW1 4RG
Tel: 020 7772 6309
http://www.rcog.org.uk/

The Royal College of Obstetricians and Gynaecologists (RCOG) states as its objectives the encouragement of the study and the advancement of the science and practice of gynaecology. The RCOG publishes a number of guidelines on the use of ultrasound in their website 'Information Services' section.

The Society and The College of Radiographers
207 Providence Square
Mill Street
London SE1 2EW

Tel: 020 7740 7200
Fax: 020 7740 7205
http://www.sor.org.news.news.htm

The Society of Radiographers includes in its objectives the promotion and development of the science and practice of radiography and radiotherapeutic technology and allied subjects. It publishes the results of study and research work therein and encourages public education, as well as protecting the honour and interests of those working in this field.

United Kingdom Association of Sonographers

36 Portland Place
London W1B 1LS
Tel: 0207 636 3714
http://www.ukasonographers.org

The United Kingdom Association of Sonographers (UKAS) produces guidelines that cover many areas, including medicolegal issues, audit and quality assurance, reporting of examinations, scanning procedures, communication to the patient and relevant clinician, ultrasound equipment usage and safe use and safety of ultrasound examination.

Useful websites

American Institute of Ultrasound in Medicine: http://www.aium.org
The American Institute of Ultrasound in Medicine is a multidisciplinary organization dedicated to advancing the art and science of ultrasound in medicine and research through its educational, scientific, literary and professional activities. The website contains a useful menu selection on 'Standards for the Performance of Ultrasound Examination'.

European Federation of Societies for Ultrasound in Medicine and Biology: http://www.efsumb.org
The Federation's purpose is to promote the exchange of scientific knowledge and development in the medical and biological professions as applied to ultrasound, proposing standards and giving advice concerning criteria for the optimum apparatus and techniques, together with presentation and interpretation of results.

World Federation of Ultrasound in Medicine and Biology: http://www.wfumb.org
WFUMB is a federation of affiliated organizations consisting of regional federations and national societies for ultrasound in medicine and biology, including the AIUM and EFSUMB mentioned above. WFUMB organizes world congresses in ultrasound every 3 years covering the whole field of diagnostic ultrasound and organizes and sponsors workshops on safety of ultrasound in medicine. Reports are published in the official journal of WFUMB, 'Ultrasound in Medicine and Biology' (UMB), published monthly by Elsevier Science Inc. See also www.elsevier.com/locate/ultrasmedbio.

http://www.omni.ac.uk and http://nmap.ac.uk/

OMNI (Organising Medical Networked Information) and NMAP (Nursing, Midwifery and the Allied Health Professions) are gateways to Internet resources in medicine, biomedicine, allied health, health management and the Social Sciences. They aim to provide comprehensive coverage of the UK resources in both areas and provide access to the best resources worldwide.

http://www.figo.org/

The International Federation of Gynecology and Obstetrics (FIGO) is a worldwide organization of obstetricians and gynaecologists. The aim of FIGO is to promote the well-being of women and to raise the standard of practice in obstetrics and gynaecology. The website provides information about FIGO's activities, events and projects, together with access to some of their publications including the FIGO newsletter, ethical guideline and annual reports.

http://209.217.125.17/SOGCnet/sogc docs/common/guide/pdfs/ps30.pdf

This website links to the Guidelines for the Performance of Ultrasound Examination in Obstetrics and Gynaecology, a policy statement prepared by the Diagnostic Imaging Committee of the Society of Obstetricians and Gynaecologists of Canada. It outlines a standard for practitioners performing ultrasound studies of the female pelvis, including routine obstetrical ultrasound, fetal sex determination and use of ultrasound in delivery room emergencies.

Further reading

The following are recommended as source reading for most aspects of obstetrics and gynaecology ultrasound. Books and articles relating to more specific aspects are listed under individual chapters.

Beischer N A, Mackay E V, Colditz P B 1997 Obstetrics and the newborn, 3rd edn. W B Saunders, London

Chudleigh P, Pearce J M 1992 Obstetric ultrasound: how, why and when. Churchill Livingstone, Edinburgh

College of Radiographers 1995 Guidance for obstetric and gynaecology ultrasound departments. White Crescent Press, Luton

Dewbury K, Meire H, Cosgrove D (eds) 1993 Ultrasound in obstetrics and gynaecology. Churchill Livingstone, Edinburgh

Dodson M G 1995 Transvaginal ultrasound, 2nd edn. Churchill Livingstone, New York

Fleisher A C, Romero R, Manning F A, Jeanty P, James A E Jr 1991 The principles and practice of ultrasonography in obstetrics and gynecology, 4th edn. Appleton & Lange, New York

Kohner N 1991 Stillbirth and Neonatal Death Society (SANDS) guidelines for professionals. Pandora, London

Neilson J P, Chambers S E (eds) 1994 Obstetric ultrasound 2. Oxford Medical Publications, Oxford

Rumack C M, Wilson S R, Charboneau J W (eds) 1998 Diagnostic ultrasound, 2nd edn. Mosby, St Louis

Sanders R C et al (eds) 1998 Clinical sonography: a practical guide, 3rd edn. Lippincott-Raven, Philadelphia

SATFA (Support around Termination for Fetal Abnormality) 1995 SATFA guidelines – ultrasonographers. Good News Press, Ongar, Essex

SATFA (Support around Termination for Fetal Abnormality) 2000 A handbook to be given to parents when an abnormality is diagnosed in their unborn baby. Good News Press Ltd, Ongar, Essex

Steel W B, Cochrane W J (eds) 1984 Gynecologic ultrasound. Clinics in diagnostic ultrasound. Churchill Livingstone, New York

United Kingdom Association of Sonographers 1995 Guidelines for professional working practice – Reporting. UKAS, London

United Kingdom Association of Sonographers 1996 Guidelines for professional working standards – Ultrasound Practice. UKAS, London

Anatomy

Scientific articles

Conner C E 1999 Scanning the fetal heart – normal appearance. BMUS Bulletin 7(2): 4–12

Dixon A N 1997 GENETICS – Made simple??! UKAS Reverberations, November: 17–19

Hay S, McLean E 1994 The timing and content of routine obstetric ultrasound in the United Kingdom. College of Radiographers, London

Gaunt M L, Beck I 1996 Imaging management of the infertile couple. BMUS Bulletin 4(1): 14–16

Ikhena S E, Konje K C 1999 Amniotic fluid volume in pregnancy: assessment and its value in the monitoring of fetal wellbeing. BMUS Bulletin, 7(1): 19–25

Whitcombe J B, Radford A 1986 Obstetric ultrasonography, a wider role for radiographers. British Medical Journal 292: 113–115

Books

Clarke K C 1973 Positioning in radiography, 9th edn. Heinemann, London
Connor J M, Ferguson-Smith M A 1991 Essential medical genetics, 3rd edn. Blackwell, Oxford
Hamilton W J (ed) 1988 Textbook of human anatomy, 2nd edn. Macmillan, London
Miller A W F, Hanretty K P 1997 Obstetrics illustrated, 5th edn. Churchill Livingstone, New York
Moore K L, Persaud T V N 1998 The developing human – clinical oriented embryology, 6th edn. W B Saunders, Philadelphia
Sharland G 2000 Cardiac abnormalities. In: Twining P, McHugo J M, Pilling D W (eds) Textbook of fetal abnormalities. Churchill Livingstone, London
Simpson J L, Golbus M S 1992 Genetics in obstetrics and gynecology, 2nd edn. W B Saunders, Philadelphia
Tortora G J, Grabowski S R 2000 Principles of anatomy and physiology, 9th edn. Wiley, New York

Physics and instrumentation

Scientific articles

American Institute of Ultrasound in Medicine (AIUM) 1988 Bioeffects considerations for the safety of diagnostic ultrasound. Journal of Ultrasound Medicine 7(9): S4
BMUS Safety Group 2000 Guidelines for the safe use of diagnostic ultrasound equipment. BMUS Bulletin 8(3): 30–33
BMUS Safety Group 2000 Statement on the safe use, and potential hazards, of diagnostic ultrasound. BMUS Bulletin 8(3): 29
Brough P 1990 Quality assurance of high resolution, real time ultrasound equipment. Radiography Today 56: 16–17
Collier D 1994 Ultrasound service contracts. BMUS Bulletin 2(1): 20–22
Cosgrove D 1995 Echo enhancers – 'contrast' agents for ultrasound. BMUS Bulletin 3(1): 34–38
Coulthard P J 1996 Quality assurance management applied to ultrasound equipment. UKAS Reverberations July: 9–13
Doody C 1997 Heating of fetal bone. BMUS Bulletin 5(4): 16–18
Dubbins P A 1992 Output power and safety – a clinical perspective. BMUS Bulletin, May: 65: 9–10
Duck F A 1992 Quantities for measurement of ultrasound exposure. BMUS Bulletin, May: 65: 14–16
Duck F A 1997 Exploring safety issues in diagnostic ultrasound. BMUS Bulletin 5(4): 4
Duck F A 2000 BMUS safety guidelines and safety statement. BMUS Bulletin 8(3): 29
European Federation of Societies for Ultrasound in Medicine and Biology 1996 Clinical safety: statement for diagnostic ultrasound. BMUS Bulletin 5(2): 20
European Federation of Societies for Ultrasound in Medicine and Biology 1996 Clinical safety: statement for diagnostic ultrasound. BMUS Bulletin 5(4): 9
European Federation of Societies for Ultrasound in Medicine and Biology 2002 Clinical safety: statement for diagnostic ultrasound. EFSUMB Newsletter 15(2): 12
European Federation of Societies for Ultrasound in Medicine and Biology 2002 Safety Committee literature reviews 2001. EFSUMB Newsletter 15(2): 13
European Federation of Societies for Ultrasound in Medicine and Biology 2002 Safety tutorial: epidemiology of diagnostic ultrasound exposure during pregnancy. EFSUMB Newsletter 16(1): 15–18
Evans D H 1998 Theory and applications of power Doppler. Reflections 3(2): 8–10
Evans T 1992 Safety in ultrasound – overview. BMUS Bulletin, May: 65: 17
Fairhead A 2000 Transvaginal scanning: what you should know about your scanner. BMUS Bulletin 8(1): 8–11

Farrell T, Leslie J, Chien P F W 2000 Three-dimensional ultrasound: reliability and validity of volumetric measurements and potential applications in obstetrics and gynaecology. BMUS Bulletin, November: 8(4): 28–35

Green V S 1995 Medico-legal issues for radiographers working in ultrasound. BMUS Bulletin 3(4): 10–22

Hartell S 2000 Purchasing ultrasound equipment. BMUS Bulletin 10(2): 54

McHugh D 1994 Quality assurance applied to ultrasound equipment. BMUS Bulletin 2(1): 25–28

Meire H 1992 Medico-legal aspects of fetal abnormality diagnosis by ultrasound. Reflections 4(1): 14–16

Merrit C R B, Kremaku F W, Hobins J C 1992 Diagnostic ultrasound: bioeffects and safety. Ultrasound Review of Obstetrics and Gynecology 2: 366–374

Mills S 1994 Ultrasound audit – the manager's view. BMUS Bulletin 2(1): 17–18

Picereing S A 1994 Equipment selection update. BMUS Bulletin 2(1): 23–24

Pilling D 1995 Retention of records in obstetrics ultrasound. BMUS Bulletin 3(1): 40

Shirrley I M 1994 Ultrasound audit clinician's view. BMUS Bulletin 2(1): 12–16

Tydeman G 2002 Digital image archiving in obstetrics – one obstetrician's perspective. BMUS Bulletin 10(1): 35–36

World Federation of Ultrasound in Medicine and Biology 1997 Statements and recommendation of safety of ultrasound in medicine. BMUS Bulletin 5(4): 6–8

Books

Barnett S B, Tor Haar G, Duck F A 2000 Guidelines and recommendation for the safe use of diagnostic ultrasound: the user's responsibility. In: Haar G T, Duck F A (eds) The safe use of ultrasound in medical diagnosis. BMUS/BIR, Alden Group, Oxford: Ch. 11

Bonilla-Musoles F, Machado L E, Osborne N G 2000 Three-dimensional ultrasound for the new millennium. Aloka Co. Ltd, Tokyo (printed in Spain)

Deane C 2000 Doppler ultrasound principles and practice. In: Nicolaides K H, Rizzo G, Hecher K (eds) Placental and fetal Doppler. Parthenon, New York

Deane C 2000 Safety of diagnostic ultrasound in fetal scanning. In: Nicolaides K H, Rizzo G, Hecher K (eds) Placental and fetal Doppler. Parthenon, New York

Evans T 1997 Principles of equipment selection. In: Bates J (ed) Practical gynaecological ultrasound. Greenwich Medical Media, London

Fish P 1990 Physics and instrumentation of diagnostic medical ultrasound. Wiley, Chichester

Haar G 2000 Bioeffects – cells and tissues. In: Haar G T, Duck F A (eds) The safe use of ultrasound in medical diagnosis. BMUS/BIR, Alden Group, Oxford: Ch. 7

Haar G T, Duck F A (eds) 2000 The safe use of ultrasound in medical diagnosis. BMUS/BIR, Alden Group, Oxford

Higashi Y, Mizushima A, Matsumoto H 1991 Introduction to abdominal ultrasonography. Springer, Berlin

McDicken W N 1991 Diagnostic ultrasonics, principles and use of instruments. Churchill Livingstone, Edinburgh

McDicken W N 1994 Purchasing ultrasonic equipment for use in obstetrics and gynaecology. In: Neilsen J P, Chambers S E (eds) Obstetric ultrasound 2. Oxford Medical Publications, Oxford

Richardson R E (ed) 1988 Guidelines for the routine performance checking of medical ultrasound equipment. Institute of Physical Sciences in Medicine, Bristol

Watson A 1996 Ultrasound equipment selection – choosing ultrasound imaging equipment. 'Which?' Ultrasound Scanner. BMUS Bulletin 4(4): 18–22

Gynaecology

Scientific articles

Bourne T 1992 Transvaginal colour Doppler sonography of the uterus and ovaries. Ultrasound in Obstetrics and Gynaecology, Schering Health Care. Fusion Communications, London

Carlin J, Thomas N B, Ludlam A E 1997 Case reports – ultrasound detection of Mirena intrauterine contraceptive devices. BMUS Bulletin 5(1): 10–13

Clewes J 1996 Ultrasound news and views. BMUS Bulletin 4(1): 38

Clewes J, Swallow J 1992 Transvaginal ultrasound in obstetrics and gynaecology – a practical guide. Ultrasound in Obstetrics and Gynaecology, Schering Health Care. Fusion Communications, London

Dagenhardt F, Jibril S, Eishenhauer B et al 1993 Vaginal hysterosalpingo – contrast sonography. BMUS Bulletin 1(4): 36–37

Deans H E, Coutts H 2000 Ovarian and adnexal pathology. BMUS Bulletin 8(2): 18–21

Epstein M 2000 Ultrasound in the management of postmenopausal bleeding (PMB). BMUS Bulletin 10(4): 18–22

Farrell T, Lesley J 2000 Three dimensional ultrasound: reliability and validity of volumetric measurements and potential applications in obstetrics and gynaecology. BMUS Bulletin 10(4): 18–22

Lakhani K P, Hardiman P 1997 Comparison of uterine artery blood flow parameters in women with dysfunctional uterine bleeding, fibroids and healthy controls. BMUS Bulletin 5(2): 25–26

Massaouh H 1993 Transvaginal sonography in gynaecology and pelvic diseases. BMUS Bulletin 1(4): 20–24

Naidoo K 2000 Transvaginal ultrasound in gynaecology – the normal and abnormal pelvis. BMUS Bulletin 8(2): 12–16

Royal College of Radiologists 1998 Intimate examinations – guidance for members and fellows, BMUS Bulletin 6(4): 50

Sanaullah F, Noran P, Louhney A D 2000 The role of ultrasound in intrapartum care. BMUS Bulletin 10(4): 23–27

Smith B 1998 Technical developments in gynaecological ultrasound. UKAS Reverberations March: 7–13

Swallow J, Clewes J 1996 The role of ultrasound in the diagnosis and treatment of female infertility. BMUS Bulletin 4(1): 18–23

Valentin L 2000 Incidental detected ovarian cysts in postmenopausal woman. BMUS Bulletin 10(4): 15–16

Books

Bates J (ed) 1997 Practical gynaecological ultrasound. Greenwich Medical Media, London

Bisset R A L, Khan A N, Thomas N B 1997 Part 2 gynaecology. In: McHugo J M (ed) Differential diagnosis in obstetric and gynecologic ultrasound. W B Saunders, London

Parsons J H, Steer C V 1993. In: Dewbury K, Meire H, Cosgrove D (eds) Ultrasound in obstetrics and gynaecology. Churchill Livingstone, Edinburgh

Yee B, Rosen G F, Cassidenti D L 1995 Transvaginal sonography in infertility. Lippincott-Raven, Philadelphia

Obstetrics – 1st trimester

Scientific articles

Anderson J E 1993 Do pregnant women know why they are having an obstetric scan? BMUS Bulletin 1(3): 36–38

Andrews H 1993 Normal first trimester appearance using trasvaginal ultrasound. BMUS Bulletin 1(3): 8–12

Arezina J, Burdock J 1997 Ectopic pregnancy cases. UKAS Reverberations, November: 17–19

Bilardo C M, Pajkrt E, De Graaf I et al 1998 Outcome of fetuses with enlarged nuchal translucency and normal karyotype. Ultrasound in Obstetrics and Gynecology 11: 401–406

College of Radiographers 1988 A code of professional conduct for radiographers. COR, London

College of Radiographers 1992 Guidelines on communication with pregnant women. Radiography Today, May: 29

Daly-Jones E 1995 There is a problem with the fetus – what do you say? BMUS Bulletin 3(1): 16

Denbow M L, Fisk N M 1996 Modern imaging in monochorionic twin pregnancies. BMUS Bulletin 4(2): 19–26

Dezateux C, Peckham C 1998 Testing times for pregnant women. Lancet (Suppl IV): 24

Dornan J C 1993 Early amniocentesis. BMUS Bulletin 1(3): 34–35
Duncan K A 2000 Transvaginal ultrasonography in early normal pregnancy. BMUS Bulletin 8(1): 12–15
Gazvani M R 2000 Ultrasonography in early pregnancy loss. BMUS Bulletin 8(1): 16–21
Gibbs V, Grime M 1999 Counselling skills for ultrasonographers – breaking bad news. BMUS Bulletin 7(4): 28–30
Goldberg H 1997 First trimester screening. UKAS Reverberations, July.
Goldberg J D 1998 Opinion. Ultrasound in Obstetrics and Gynecology 12: 6–7
Harrington K, Tunbel S, Campbell S 1993 Screening for fetal anomalies with transvaginal ultrasound in early pregnancy. BMUS Bulletin 1(34): 13–17
Hyde B 1986 An interview study of pregnant women's attitude to ultrasound scanning. Social Science and Medicine 22(5): 587–592
Jones T 2001 National guidelines on early pregnancy scanning. BMUS Bulletin 9(1): 12
Liu D T Y 1993 Controversies in ultrasound. 1st trimester karyotype – how should we do it? Chorion villus sampling – current utility and future potential. BMUS Bulletin 1(3): 31–33
Neales K 1996 Multiple pregnancy – clinical aspects of management. BMUS Bulletin 4(2): 4–12
Smith A P M 1996 The role of ultrasound in twin pregnancies. BMUS Bulletin 4(2): 13–18
Smith J, Smith A P M 1995 Obstetric ultrasound: psychological dimension. BMUS Bulletin 3(6): 25–26
Smulian J C, Egan J F X, Rodis J F 1998 Fetal hydrops in the first trimester associated with maternal parvovirus infection. Journal of Clinical Ultrasound 26(6): July/August: 314–316
Snidjers R J M, Noble P, Sebire N et al 1998 UK multicentre project on assessment of risk of trisomy 21 by maternal age and fetal nuchal translucency thickness at 10–14 weeks of gestation. Lancet 352: 343–346
Souka A P, Nicolaides K H 1997 Diagnosis of fetal abnormalities at the 10–14 week scan. Ultrasound in Obstetrics and Gynecology 10: 429–442
Souka A P, Snidjers R J M, Novakov A et al 1998 Defects and syndromes in chromosomal normal fetuses with increased nuchal translucency thickness at 10–14 weeks of gestation. Ultrasound in Obstetrics and Gynecology 11: 391–400
Speck R P 1991 Breaking bad news. Nursing Times 87(12): 24–26
Starrs L, Burnside A 1998 Caring for those who miscarry. UKAS Reverberations, March: 2–5
Stirrat G 1998 Acknowledging pregnancy loss – hydatidiform mole. The Miscarriage Association, Wakefield
Tasker M, Booth A 1998 Nuchal translucency in a fetus with Zellweger's syndrome. BMUS Bulletin: 6(2) 26
Twinning P The first trimester diagnosis of fetal abnormalities. BMUS Bulletin 8(2): 22–30
United Kingdom Association of Sonographers 1995 Guidelines for professional working practice – reporting. UKAS, London
United Kingdom Association of Sonographers 1996 Guidelines for professional working standards – ultrasound practice. UKAS, London
Van Os H C, Hout J, Janson C A M 1993 Embryonic length, crown-rump length and fetal heart activity in early human pregnancy determination by transvaginal ultrasound. BMUS Bulletin 1(3): 18–23
Whitcombe J B, Radford A 1986 Obstetric ultrasonography, a wider role for radiographers. British Medical Journal 292: 113–115

Books

Cacciatore B 1994 Ectopic pregnancy; imaging and modern concepts of management. In: Neilson J P, Chambers S E (eds) Obstetric ultrasound 2. Oxford Medical Publications, Oxford
Callen H L 1988 Ultrasonography in obstetrics and gynecology. 2nd edn. W B Saunders, Philadelphia
Cochrane W J 1985 Ultrasound and the intrauterine device. In: Sanders R C, James A E (eds) The principles and practice of ultrasonography in obstetrics and gynecology, 3rd edn. Appleton-Century-Crofts, Norwalk, Connecticut

Kaplan P M 1991 Intrauterine contraceptive device. In: Sanders R C (ed) Clinical sonography. Little, Brown, Boston

Keit J 2000 Now you've found two, what should you do? A question of chorionicity. UKAS Reverberations March: 7–8

Lyons E A, Levi C S, Dashefsky S M 1998 The first trimester. In: Rumach C M, Wilson S R, Charboneau J M (eds) Diagnostic ultrasound, 2nd edn. Mosby, St Louis

Miscarriage Association 1998 Acknowledging pregnancy loss – the hidden grief. Coping with miscarriage. RAP Ltd, Rochdale

Miscarriage Association 1998 Acknowledging pregnancy loss – why did this happen to us? A summary of causes, tests and treatment, RAP Ltd, Rochdale

Moore K L, Persaud T V N 1998 The developing human – clinical oriented embryology, 6th edn. W B Saunders, Philadelphia

Nicolaides K H, Sebire N J, Snidjers R J M 1999 The 11–14 week scan. The diagnosis of fetal abnormalities. Parthenon, New York

Nyerberg D A 1990 Diagnostic ultrasound of fetal anomalies: text and atlas. Year Book, Chicago

Sanders R C, Blackmon L R, Hogge W A, Wulfsberg E A (eds) 1996 Structural fetal abnormalities – the total picture. Mosby, St Louis

Snidjers R J M, Nicolaides K H 1996 Ultrasound markers for fetal chromosomal defects. Parthenon, New York

Twining P 2000 First trimester detection of fetal anomalies. In: Twining P, McHugo J M, Pilling D W (eds) Textbook of fetal abnormalities. Churchill Livingstone, London

Walker J 1998 Acknowledging pregnancy loss – ectopic pregnancy. The Miscarriage Association, Wakefield

Obstetrics – 2nd and 3rd trimester, part one

Scientific articles

Allan D 1992 Doppler ultrasound in medicine Part 2; clinical applications. Hospital Update, April.

Allen A L, Feely A, McInnes E 1997 Case report. Reflections on the need for sonographer awareness of possible consequences of liver disease in pregnancy. BMUS Bulletin 5(4): 45–47

Bleakney R R, Duncan K A 2001 Antenatal hydronephrosis – neonatal follow up. BMUS Bulletin 9(1): 23–27

Brennand J E, Macara L M 1999 Fetal heart – abnormal appearances. BMUS Bulletin 7(2): 14–19

Chamberlain P 1992 Composite sonographic assessment of fetal health. Current Opinion in Obstetrics and Gynaecology 4: 256–263

Chiswik M L 1985 Intrauterine growth retardation. British Medical Journal 291: 845

Chitty L Y N 1994 Charts of fetal size. BMUS Bulletin 2(4): 9–19

College of Radiographers 1988 A code of professional conduct for radiographers. COR, London

College of Radiographers 1992 Guidelines on communication with pregnant women. Radiography Today, May: 29

Conner C E 1999 Scanning the fetal heart – normal appearance. BMUS Bulletin 7(2): 4–12

Denbow M L, Fisk N M 1996 Modern imaging in monochorionic twin pregnancies. BMUS Bulletin 4(2): 19–24

Department of Health 1995 The patient's charter and maternity services. DoH, London

Douilet P M, Benson C B 1990 Fetal growth disturbances. Seminars in Roentgenology XXV(4): 309–316

European Federation of Societies for Ultrasound in Medicine and Biology 2001 Diagnostic amniocentesis in singleton pregnancy: guidelines suggested by EFSUMB's Educational and Professional Standards Committee. EFSUMB Newsletter 14(2): 6–8

Fleishcher A, Guidetti D, Stuhlmuller P 1989 Umbilical artery velocity waveforms in the intrauterine growth retarded fetus. Clinical Obstetrics and Gynaecology 329(4): 660–668

Gardener G, Chitty L 2001 Prenatal diagnosis of cystic lung lesions. BMUS Bulletin 9(2): 8–13

Gardosi J 1994 Customised fetal growth charts. BMUS Bulletin 2(4): 20–24

Hyde B 1986 An interview study of pregnant women's attitude to ultrasound scanning. Social Science and Medicine 22(5): 587–592

Ikhena S E, Konje K C 1999 Amniotic fluid volume in pregnancy: assessment and its value in the monitoring of fetal wellbeing. BMUS Bulletin 7(1): 19–25

James D 1990 Diagnosis and management of fetal growth retardation. Archives of Disease in Childhood 65: 390–394

Jeffrey F, Peipert J F, Donnenfeld A E 1991 Oligohydramnios: a review. Obstetrical and Gynecological Survey 46(6): 325–339

Jones A, Cook A, Simpson J 2002 Prenatal detection of congenital heart disease: identification of high-risk groups and normal sonographic appearances. BMUS Bulletin 10(1): 6–10

Kurjak A, Zmijanac J 1992 Management of the growth retarded fetus. Clinical Obstetrics and Gynaecology 35(1): 185–193

Lim B H 2000 Transvaginal ultrasound – applications in the second and third trimesters of pregnancy. BMUS Bulletin 8(1): 22–25

Masturzo B, Chitty L 2001 Hyperechogenic kidneys in the fetus: diagnosis and management. BMUS Bulletin 9(2): 22–27

Neales K 1996 Multiple pregnancy – clinical aspects of management. BMUS Bulletin 4(2): 4–12

Royal College of Obstetricians and Gynaecologists 1984 Routine ultrasound examination in pregnancy. RCOG, London

Smith A P M 1996 The role of ultrasound in twin pregnancies. BMUS Bulletin 1(4): 25–35

Twining P 1995 Oligohydramnios – current thoughts and a diagnostic review. BMUS Bulletin 3(2): 30–32

Valentin L, Hackeloer J 2001 Diagnostic amniocentesis in singleton pregnancies. Guidelines suggested by the European Federation of Societies for Ultrasound in Medicine and Biology Educational and Professional Standards Committee. EFSUMB Newsletter 14(2): 6–8

Valentin L, Jensen S S 2002 Diagnostic chorionic villus sampling (CVS) in singleton pregnancies. EFSUMB Newsletter 16(1): 8–11

Walkinshaw S A 2001 Minor markers and aneuploidy. BMUS Bulletin 9(1): 19–22

Warshaw J B 1991 Nutritional perturbation in infants of diabetic mothers and intrauterine growth retardation. Seminars in Perinatology 15(6): 456–461

Watt J 1989 The consequences of intrauterine growth retardation: what do we know? Australian and New Zealand Journal of Obstetrics and Gynaecology 29(3 Pt 2): 279–287

Whittle M J 1990 Imaging problems in obstetrics. Clinical Physics and Physiological Measurement 11(Suppl A): 109–111

Wilde P 1996 Fetal echocardiography. UKAS Reverberations, July: 5–8

Zimmer E Z, Divon M Y 1992 Sonographic diagnosis of IUGR – macrosomia. Clinical Obstetrics and Gynaecology 35(1): 172–184

Books

ATL Ultrasound 1999 Obstetrics and gynecology ultrasound protocol guides. ATL Ultrasound, Bothwell, Washington

Chamberlain G (ed) 1990 Modern antenatal care of the fetus. Blackwell Scientific, Oxford

Chudleigh T, Cook K 2001 Cleft lip and palate – a guide for sonographers. Cleft Lip and Palate Association, London.

Deter R L, Hadlock F P, Harrist R B 1983 Evaluation of normal foetal growth retardation. In: Callen P (ed) Ultrasonography in obstetrics and gynaecology. W B Saunders, Philadelphia

Fong K W, Farine D 1998 Cervical incompetence and preterm labour. In: Rumack C M, Wilson S R, Charboneau J W (eds) Diagnostic ultrasound, 2nd edn. Mosby, St Louis

Huggon I C 2001 Practical guide to fetal echocardiography. In: Prenatal and neonatal medicine, Vol. 6, No. 1. Parthenon, New York

Kane R 1986 The cervical stitch: what it's like. The Miscarriage Association. Algate Press, Wakefield

Kurtz A B, Middleton W D 1996 Ultrasound – the requisites. Mosby, St Louis

Landers D V, Sweet R L 1992 Infectious agents. In: Simpson J L, Golbus M S (eds) Genetics in obstetrics and gynaecology, 2nd edn. W B Saunders, Philadelphia

Llewellyn-Jones D 1990 Fundamentals of obstetrics and gynaecology, 5th edn. Faber & Faber, London

Manning F A, Holder C 1991 Intrauterine growth retardation: diagnosis, prognostication, and management based on ultrasound methods. In: Fleischer A C, Romero R, Manning F A, Jeanty

P, James A E Jr (eds) The principles and practice of ultrasonography in obstetrics and gynaecology, 4th edn. Appleton & Lange, New York

Pilu G, Nicolaides K H 1999 Diagnosis of fetal abnormalities – the 18–23 week scan. Parthenon, London

Royal College of Obstetricians and Gynaecologists 1996 Termination of pregnancy for fetal abnormality – in England, Wales and Scotland. RCOG, London

Sanders R C, Blackmon L R, Hogge W A, Wulfsberg E A (eds) 1996 Structural fetal abnormalities – the total picture. Mosby, St Louis

Simpson J L, Golbus M S 1992 Genetics in obstetrics and gynecology, 2nd edn. W B Saunders, Philadelphia

Snidjers R J M, Nicolaides K H 1996 Ultrasound markers for fetal chromosomal defects. Parthenon, New York

Obstetrics – 2nd and 3rd trimester, part two

Scientific articles

Allan D 1992 Doppler ultrasound in medicine. Part 2: clinical applications. Hospital Update, April

Chamberlain P 1992 Composite sonographic assessment of fetal health. Current Opinion in Obstetrics and Gynaecology 4: 256–263

Chiswik M L 1985 Intrauterine growth retardation. British Medical Journal 291: 845

Chitty L Y N 1994 Charts of fetal size. BMUS Bulletin 2(4): 9–19

Chitty L, Altman D 2001 Charts of fetal size. In: Dewbury K et al (eds) clinical ultrasound – a comprehensive text – ultrasound in obstetrics and gynaecology, 2nd edn.

Clark T J, Dwarakanath L, Weaver J B 1999 Pruritus in pregnancy and obstetric cholestasis (review). Hospital Medicine 60(4): 254–260

College of Radiographers 1992 Guidelines on communication with pregnant women. Radiography Today, May: 29

Denbow M L, Fisk N M 1996 Modern imaging in monochorionic twin pregnancies. BMUS Bulletin 4(2): 19–26

Department of Health 1995 The patient's charter and maternity services. DoH, London

Douilet P M, Benson C B 1990 Fetal growth disturbances. Seminars in Roentgenology XXV(4): 309–316

Fleischcer A, Guidetti D, Stuhlmuller P 1989 Umbilical artery velocity waveforms in the intrauterine growth retarded fetus. Clinical Obstetrics and Gynaecology 329(4): 660–668

Green M 1999 Transabdominal versus transvaginal ultrasound for placenta previa. UKAS Reverberations, July: 6–8

Heinonen S, Kirkien P 1999 Pregnancy outcome with intrahepatic cholestasis. Obstetrics and Gynecology 94(2): 189–193

Hyde B 1986 An interview study of pregnant women's attitude to ultrasound scanning. Social Science and Medicine 22(5): 587–592

Ikhena S E, Konje J C 1999 Amniotic fluid volume in pregnancy: assessment and its value in the monitoring of fetal wellbeing. BMUS Bulletin: (1): 19–25

James D 1990 Diagnosis and management of fetal growth retardation. Archives of Disease in Childhood 65: 390–394

Jones A, Cook A, Simpson J 2002 Prenatal detection of congenital heart disease: identification of high-risk groups and normal sonographic appearances. BMUS Bulletin 10(1): 6–10

Kurjak A, Zmijanac J 1992 Management of the growth retarded fetus. Clinical Obstetrics and Gynaecology 35(1): 185–193

Loughna P 2000 Doppler of fetal venous circulation. BMUS Bulletin 10(4): 6–8

Matos A, Bernardes J, Ayres-de-Campos D, Patricio B 1997 Antepartum fetal cerebral hemorrhage not predicted by current surveillance methods in cholestasis of pregnancy. Obstetrics and Gynecology 89(5 Pt 2): 803–804

McDonald J A 1999 Cholestasis of pregnancy (review). Journal of Gastroenterology and Hepatology 14(6): 515–518

Neales K 1996 Multiple pregnancy – clinical aspects of management. BMUS Bulletin 4(2): 4–12

Papageorghiou A T, Bower S 2000 Second trimester uterine artery Doppler screening for placental insufficiency. BMUS Bulletin 10(4): 10–12

Reyes H 1997 Intrahepatic cholestasis: a puzzling disorder of pregnancy (review). Journal of Gastroenterology and Hepatology 12(3): 211–216

Smith A P M 1996 The role of ultrasound in twin pregnancies. BMUS Bulletin 4(2): 13–17

Turner G M, Twining P 1994 The antenatal diagnosis of skeletal dysplasias: a simplified approach. BMUS Bulletin 2(4): 32–38

Twining P 1995 Oligohydramnios – current thoughts and a diagnostic review. BMUS Bulletin 3(2): 30–33

Warshaw J B 1991 Nutritional perturbation in infants of diabetic mothers and intrauterine growth retardation. Seminars in Perinatology 15(6): 456–461

Watt J 1989 The consequences of intrauterine growth retardation: what do we know? Australian and New Zealand Journal of Obstetrics and Gynaecology 29(3 Pt 2): 279–287

Whittle M J 1990 Imaging problems in obstetrics. Clinical Physics and Physiological Measurement 11(Suppl A): 109–111

Zimmer E Z, Divon M Y 1992 Sonographic diagnosis of IUGR – macrosomia. Clinical Obstetrics and Gynaecology 35(1): 172–184

Books

Bisset R A L, Khan A N, Thomas N B 1997 Part 1 obstetrics. In: McHugo J M (ed) Differential diagnosis in obstetric and gynecologic ultrasound. W B Saunders, London

Chamberlain G (ed) 1990 Modern antenatal care of the fetus. Blackwell Scientific, Oxford

College of Radiographers 1988 A code of professional conduct for radiographers. COR, London

Deter R L, Hadlock F P, Harrist R B 1983 Evaluation of normal foetal growth retardation. In: Callen P (ed) Ultrasonography in obstetrics and gynaecology. W B Saunders, Philadelphia

Fong K W, Farine D 1998 Cervical incompetence and preterm labour. In: Rumack C M, Wilson S R, Charboneau J W (eds) Diagnostic ultrasound, 2nd edn. Mosby, St Louis

Kane R 1986 The cervical stitch: what it's like. The Miscarriage Association. Algate Press, Wakefield

Landers D V, Sweet R L 1992 Infectious agents. In: Simpson J L, Golbus M S (eds) Genetics in obstetrics and gynaecology, 2nd edn. W B Saunders, Philadelphia

Llewellyn-Jones D, Abraham S, Oats J (eds) 1999 Fundamentals of obstetrics and gynaecology, 7th edn. Mosby, London

Manning F A, Holder C 1991 Intrauterine growth retardation: diagnosis, prognostication, and management based on ultrasound methods. In: Fleischer A C, Romero R, Manning F A, Jeanty P, James A E Jr (eds) The principles and practice of ultrasonography in obstetrics and gynaecology, 4th edn. Appleton & Lange, New York

Nicolaides K H, Rizzo G, Hecher K 2000 Placental and fetal Doppler. Parthenon, New York

Pilu G, Nicolaides K H 1999 Diagnosis of fetal abnormalities – the 18–23 week scan. Parthenon, London

Royal College of Obstetricians and Gynaecologists 1984 Routine ultrasound examination in pregnancy. RCOG, London

Royal College of Obstetricians and Gynaecologists 1996 Termination of pregnancy for fetal abnormality – in England, Wales and Scotland. RCOG, London

Sanders R C, Blackmon L R, Hogge W A, Wulfsberg E A (eds) 1996 Structural fetal abnormalities – the total picture. Mosby, St Louis

Simpson J L, Golbus M S (eds) Genetics in obstetrics and gynaecology, 2nd edn. W B Saunders, Philadelphia

Snidjers R J M, Nicolaides K H 1996 Ultrasound markers for fetal chromosomal defects. Parthenon, New York

Spirit B A, Gordon L P 1998 Sonographic evaluation of the placenta. In: Rumack C M, Wilson S R, Charboneau J W (eds) Diagnostic ultrasound, 2nd edn. Mosby, St Louis

Stamm E R, Drose J A 1998 The fetal heart. In: Rumack C M, Wilson S R, Charboneau J W (eds) Diagnostic ultrasound, 2nd edn. Mosby, St Louis

United Kingdom Association of Ultrasonographers (UKAS) 1996 Guidelines for professional working standards – ultrasound practice. UKAS, London

Weller B F, Wells R J 1990 Baillière's Nurses Dictionary, 21st edn. Baillière Tindall, London

Yee B, Rosen G F, Cassidenti D L 1995 Transvaginal sonography in infertility. Lippincott-Raven, Philadelphia

Fertility

Scientific articles

Anon 1998 Latex sensitisation – what causes it and what can be done to minimise the risks: Part 2. Nursing Times 94(Suppl 8): 1–4

Akman M A, Garcia J E, Damewood M D et al 1996 Hydrosalpinx affects the implantation of previously cryopreserved embryos. Human Reproduction 11(5): 1013–1014

Blazar A S, Hogan J W, Seifer D B et al 1997 The impact of hydrosalpinx on successful pregnancy in tubal factor infertility treated by in vitro fertilization. Fertility and Sterility 67(3): 517–520

Clewes J 1996 Ultrasound news and views. BMUS Bulletin 4(1): 38

Cottle C 1991 Infertility: the emotional aspects. Nursing Standard 5(28): 29–31

Denbow M L, Fisk M N 1996 Modern imaging in monochorionic twin pregnancies. BMUS Bulletin 4(2): 19–26

Fleming C, Hull M G 1996 Impaired implantation after in vitro fertilisation treatment associated with hydrosalpinx. British Journal of Obstetrics and Gynaecology 103(3): 268–272

Gaunt M L, Beck I 1996 Imaging management of the infertile couple. BMUS Bulletin 4(1): 14–16

Goswany R 1992 Hysterosalpingo-contrast sonography to assess tubal patency. Ultrasound in Obstetrics and Gynaecology, Schering Health Care. Fusion Communications, London

Green S, Fishel S, Thornton S, Dowell K 1996. Assisted reproduction techniques for managing infertility. BMUS Bulletin 4(1): 4–12

Kan A K, Abdalla H I, Gafar A H et al 1999 Embryo transfer: ultrasound-guided versus clinical touch. Human Reproduction 14(5): 1259–1261

Kennedy E 1996 The impact of subfertility. BMUS Bulletin 4(1): 24–25

Krysiewicz S 1992 Infertility in women: diagnostic evaluation with hysterosalpingography and other imaging techniques. American Journal of Roentgenology 159: 253–261

Mukherjee T, Copperman A B, McCaffrey C et al 1996 Hydrosalpinx fluid has embryotoxic effects on murine embryogenesis: a case for prophylactic salpingectomy. Fertility and Sterility 66(5): 851–853

Neales K 1996 Multiple pregnancy – clinical aspects of management. BMUS Bulletin 4(2): 6–12

Omigbodun A O, Fatukasi J I, Abudu T 1992 Ultrasonography as an adjunct to hydrotubation in the management of female infertility. Central African Journal of Medicine 38(8): 345–350

Smith A P M 1996 The role of ultrasound in twin pregnancies. BMUS Bulletin 4(2): 13–18

Strandell A, Waldenstrom U, Nilsson L, Hamberger L 1994 Hydrosalpinx reduces in-vitro fertilization/embryo transfer pregnancy rates. Human Reproduction 9(5): 861–863

Swallow J, Clewes J 1996 The role of ultrasound in the diagnosis and treatment of the female infertility. BMUS Bulletin 4(1): 18–23

Tufekci E C, Girit S, Bayirli E, Durmusoglu F, Yalti S 1992 Evaluation of tubal patency by transvaginal sonosalpingography. Fertility and Sterility 57(2): 336–340

Waters J 1997 Latex gloves: still a serious occupational hazard. Nursing Times 93(25): 56–58

Waterstone J 1992 Investigation of subfertility. The Practitioner 236: 141–144

Books

Power M 1997 Fertility problems. In: Andrews G (ed) Fertility problems in women's sexual health. Baillière Tindall, London

Sanders R C 1991 Infertility diagnosis by ultrasound. Urologic radiology. Springer, New York

Wikland M 1992 Vaginal ultrasound in assisted reproduction. Baillière's Clinical Obstetrics and Gynaecology 6(2): 283–296

Yee B, Rosen G F, Cassidenti D L 1995 Transvaginal sonography in infertility. Lippincott-Raven, Philadelphia

Index